Gypsy Folk Medicine

★ ★ ★

Wanja von Hausen

Illustrated by Marlene Ekman

 Sterling Publishing Co., Inc.   New York

Illustrated by Marlene Ekman

Translated from the German by Elisabeth Reinersmann
Translation edited by Jeanette Green

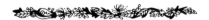

Library of Congress Cataloging-in-Publication Data

Hausen, Wanja von.
   [Geheimen Rezepte der Zigeunermedizin. English]
   Gypsy folk medicine / Wanja von Hausen.
      p.   cm.
   Translation of: Die Geheimen Rezepte der Zigeunermedizin.
   Includes index.
   ISBN 0-8069-8432-5
   1. Gypsies—Medicine. I. Title.
DX157.H3813   1991
615.8′82′08991497—dc20   91-15479
                                             CIP

10 9 8 7 6 5 4 3 2 1

English translation © 1992 by Sterling Publishing Company
Illustrations © 1992 by Sterling Publishing Company
387 Park Avenue South, New York, N.Y. 10016
Original edition published under the title *Geheimen Rezepte
der Zigeunermedizin*
© 1987 by Verlag Orac GesmbH & Co.
Distributed in Canada by Sterling Publishing
% Canadian Manda Group, P.O. Box 920, Station U
Toronto, Ontario, Canada M8Z 5P9
Distributed in Great Britain and Europe by Cassell PLC
Villiers House, 41/47 Strand, London WC2N 5JE, England
Distributed in Australia by Capricorn Link Ltd.
P.O. Box 665, Lane Cove, NSW 2066
Printed in the United States
All rights reserved

Sterling ISBN 0-8069-8432-5

CONTENTS

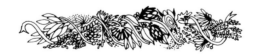

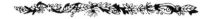

Warning

Although many species in the plant kingdom have miraculous healing properties, some are poisonous. (Mistletoe berries and jimsonweed in particular have been so considered.) Also, some plants may cause severe allergic reactions. Exercise caution in trying out any of these recipes, and consult a physician for any serious ailment.

Although a German pharmacist carefully examined the traditional folk medicine recipes in this book, their effectiveness or safety can in no way be guaranteed.

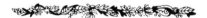

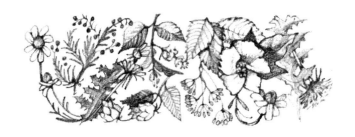

PREFACE

Pharmacist Helmut Wenning tested the recipes in this book and found them pharmacologically effective.

I have to admit, I was at first very skeptical. After all, I am a registered, certified pharmacologist, with an education based in the natural sciences. I have spent a great deal of time in research and development. To be honest, I stood solidly on the side of allopathic medicine.

However, over time I became concerned about the growing number of desperate people who came to me for help. The people who poured out their hearts suffered mostly from chronic illnesses. They had been given so many different medicines, each one praised as better or more effective. These medicines were taken in the hope that the latest one would make them well. But they were disappointed time and again. There seemed to be no escape from their cycle of illness, hope, experimentation, and failure.

One evening I visited friends in the town of Rosenheim. During that visit I met Wanja von Hausen, the author. She had just returned—all excited—from a trip to Spain and meeting with Pilar.

Ms. von Hausen gave me these Gypsy recipes for evaluation. I took much time and care testing them and found most of them quite good. Some of my pharmacy customers tried them and managed to regain their health.

On my recommendation a few traditional Gypsy remedies or particular ingredients were excluded from this book, because they should not be used in light of today's knowledge. For example, the ingredients for a salve, Bride of the Sun, lists goat butter as a base. I suggest using a more neutral base. (However, in spite of its offensive odor, goat butter does have astringent properties.)

I am convinced that synthetic substances do not have the same effects as those provided by nature, although we have been taught otherwise. Maybe Pilar is right when she insists that synthetic substances do not possess the spark of real life.

I believe all human beings have a mystical bent, even those of us who do not share this belief in elemental nature. It is of utmost importance that we trust and believe in the medicine designed to help us get well, provided we do not take a medicine that has severe side effects. We should avoid harmful drugs as long as there are natural remedies—in harmony with nature—available that may restore our health.

—HELMUT WENNING

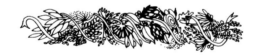

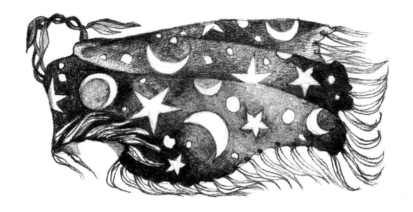

1
BATI PURÍ PILAR

"You fly to the moon, but you do not know what life is all about."

Pilar's shoulders are covered by a midnight blue shawl, embroidered with shining silvery moons. Her hair is in shiny black braids. She tilts her wicker chair, leaning against her trailer.

"Where do Gypsies come from? Some believe we are the last survivors of Atlantis. When the continent sank we were supposedly scattered all over the world. Others suggest that our ancestors are the people of the biblical town of Babel. When the Tower of Babel was destroyed, people were cursed with a confusing multitude of languages."

"Well, which is it then?" I ask.

Pilar smiles. "Choose what you wish; we don't care. What difference would it make in our lives if we knew where we came from? What, indeed, do *you* know about yourself?"

She shakes her head almost imperceptibly and reaches for a long wooden spoon with which she begins to stir soup, cooking in a belly-shaped pot that hangs over a small wood fire. She adds a twig of flowering rosemary to the soup.

"You are funny people, you *Payos*. You think by writing down, analyzing, labeling, and counting everything, you are also controlling everything, and everything is in its proper place! And what have you done to this beautiful world, to our planet? You fly to the moon, but you do not know what life is all about."

Pilar spoke in Spanish, rolling her *r*s and never raising her soft voice. She meant no ill when she called me *Paya*, a name for non-Gypsies. (*Payos*, the Romani term, means "foreigners"; *Payo* is male and *Paya* female. The English term for non-Gypsies is *Gachi* or *Gaje*.)

Gypsies are an amazing people—the only group of people living in every corner of the earth without the benefits of power, money, armies, or ever fighting a war. Wherever you travel—to the plains of Hungary, the steppes of Siberia, the gates of Marrakesh, the highlands of Guatemala, or the frozen tundra of Alaska—everywhere, except southeast Asia, you'll find Gypsies. They are always on the move and have an ever-abiding need for freedom and independence. Although many Gypsies do not read or write (their migratory way of life makes fixed-place schooling difficult), they readily master the language of their host country. Although Gypsies have occasional contact with the outside world, they prefer to remain in independent communities. No government and no monarch has been able to break the Gypsy spirit—not with gifts of land and seeds, and not with brutal persecution.

This persecution began as early as the 14th century in Romania, where Gypsies were enslaved. In 1417 census-takers first formally registered the presence of exotic strangers in Europe, and Gypsies were first denounced as enemies of Christendom. Until recently, they were considered outlaws, tortured, hanged, sold as slaves, and burned at the stake. Nazis systematically rounded them up and sent them to concentration camps, just like the Jews, to be murdered in the gas chambers.

The worldwide Gypsy population is estimated to be about twelve million. Gypsies, who call themselves Rom, originated from India. In about 1000 AD these Indians served in an army sent to fight the spread of Islam in northern India. In 1760 linguists first traced their native language, Romani, to Indian roots. Spanish Gypsies, *Gitanos*, speak Spanish with a sprinkling of Romani words, a dialect called Caló. Gitanos make up the largest minority group in Spain.

When asked about the Gypsy population worldwide, Pilar responds: "What good would it do to know the exact number of Gypsies? We see ourselves as the salt of the earth."

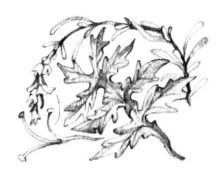

In a gentle, quiet voice—surrounded by soft, warm air on a June night on the banks of the Ebro River, where screech owls call from the nearby forest—the wise old woman tries to explain what distinguishes Gypsies from other people.

"We love the earth and we want to experience her beauty again every day. But we do not need or want to subject her to our will. We only take what she gives us freely and abundantly."

Pilar is the *Bati Purí* of her clan, (literally "Old Mother" in Romani) the wise one, the healer. No decision is made by the elected head of the clan without consulting Bati Purí Pilar. This age-old tradition is practiced in Gypsy communities worldwide. By the way, no kings or queens ever existed in Gypsy culture. That is a fantasy that lives only in the pretty world of the operetta.

The clan leader, however, has absolute power within the clan and over all clan members who elected him or her. The stories, often told by Gypsies themselves, that they are the descendants of a royal house in Asia Minor, are part of a survival philosophy. They play upon the piano of laws and ideas of their host country—staying within legal boundaries and accommodating people's expectations—as long as they do not have to sacrifice too much of their own identity. "If *Payos* dream of a duke from the Nile? Okay, we will deliver. If they want to see a Gypsy wedding? Why not perform for them what they want—for a fee, of course. After all, Gypsies have to live, too."

This is why the Gitanos in Spain and France were baptized and became Catholics. Their brothers in Morocco became Muslims; those living in northern Germany and Scandinavia became Lutherans. These public confessions made life easier for them and did not cost much.

Pilar continues: "We believe that *Undebel*, God, and *Beng*, the Devil, are in constant competition. Often it seems that Beng is gaining the upper hand. But we hope that in the end Undebel will win, after all. Don't all religions, in one form or another, believe and teach this?"

Pilar refuses to divulge anything more about Gypsy myths. Their secrets belong to them alone. Even when tortured, Gypsies did not give away their most cherished and holy secrets. Until recently, even the Catholic priest who celebrated Mass was excluded from their famous annual meeting at the Pilgrimage Church of Saint-Maries-de-la-Mer in the Camargue in the South of France.

"Don't ask any more questions."

Pilar's face tells me that I have reached the boundary no Payo is allowed to cross.

"I will entrust you with something valuable and positive."

"And what would that be?" I ask.

"The secret recipes of my healing art."

I feel as if I had just received an unexpected marriage proposal. I am bewildered, flattered, uncertain, and happy.

"What have I done to deserve this?" I ask.

"Kismet," she says. "Fate, destiny. I saw on your forehead a sign from the heavens. Yesterday."

Yesterday I brought Pilar a young boy I had found, almost lifeless, who had been hit by a car. The young boy turned out to be her great-grandson. By chance I found the injured boy in a ditch by the road, on my trip through northeastern Spain to Tortosa. When searching for a physician, I discovered twenty-seven trailers on the bank of the Ebro River.

Today, the little boy—who had been unconscious when I left him with his family yesterday—sat in a puddle, happily playing with his black and white speckled dog.

"Stay," Pilar says, following my gaze. "Write down what has never been recorded before. A girl I had entrusted with this knowledge who was one of us has disappeared. I believe we are all running out of time on this planet. We human beings, no matter where we come from, must get together and save whatever we can."

As I run to my car to get a note pad, I hear the bright and happy voice of Pilar's great-grandson, Rodrigo: "Still more questions?" He chuckles. "Nobody knows where we came from. Nobody knows where we are going!"

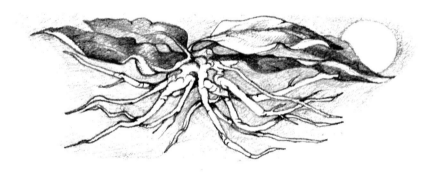

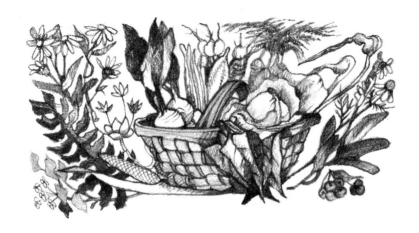

───2───
THE ART OF HEALING

"In the truest sense, a *healer* must have a deep and abiding respect for creation—for Mother Earth and for life everywhere, in all its variety."

Bati Purí Pilar sighs and reaches for a small branch that has fallen from an olive tree, and begins to draw circles and signs in the sand. For the first time I notice dark shadows under her eyes. I also notice how this wise, intelligent woman pulls her shoulders together, as if to protect herself. As if—with her promise to tell me the most secret knowledge of her people—she had embarked on a dangerous journey, she were about to balance on the edge of a cliff, or she had walked onto very thin ice over deep waters.

With a soft, sometimes hesitating voice, Pilar introduces me to a magical world—a world as she knows and experiences it. I listen and record; I try to avoid interrupting her with questions.

"An external manifestation is only part of the reality of an object or a person. Every human being, every animal, every plant possesses a unique and specific aura; even minerals have an aura. When I walk through the woods I can feel the contact that exists between trees, plants, animals, and rocks. I know if a place has positive or negative vibrations. The vibrations are not always the same. They are influenced by the sun, the moon, and the stars."

Pilar, taking a sip of red wine, looks at me with a smile, and then shrugs her shoulders.

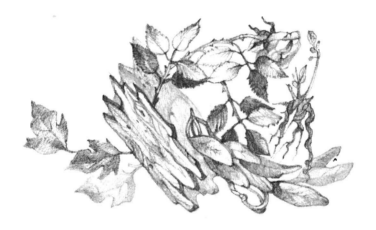

"Whenever I collect herbs, I talk to them intensely but quietly; I involve my whole being in the process of gathering. I turn to them, asking for their help. If one plant should refuse, I turn to the next plant and try to find sympathy. Because I know that if a plant does not want to give itself to me of its own free will, it will use its defense mechanism. If torn from its base, it will seal off most of its positive energy and will, therefore, only make a fraction of its potential effectiveness available to me.

"I would never tear a plant out of the ground just to throw it away afterwards. I gather only those leaves and flowers, take only those portions of a root, a bark, and fruits, that I really need. I could not sleep if I were not sure that the part of a

14

plant necessary for its survival was left intact. If I need every part of the herb (leaves, blossoms, stems, and roots), I leave the strongest portion of the plant in the ground. In that way I know that new growth is assured.

"After I have taken what I was allowed, I thank the plant for the gift it has given me. I promise the plants that my thoughts will be with them and their efforts to keep our planet alive.

"If you look intently, you will be able to detect how uniquely different one leaf is from another, one flower from another, and one tree of the same species is from another. Each living entity—human being, animal, plant—has its own individuality. And only that which is alive can create life.

"Scientists think that when they have analyzed and separated something into chemical components they have discovered its secret. I think the opposite is true.

"Because no matter how many 'ingredients' they create and mix together, no matter how long they try—they cannot create life, because they cannot create the spark of life.

"If I eat a lemon or take synthetically produced vitamin C it makes a difference, just as the bark of a willow tree [which contains salicylic acid] is more effective against pain than over-the-counter salicylic acid [aspirin].

"Always remember the person's inviolable individuality when you try my recipes for healing. Observe the person's reaction. Don't forget that the person does not just suffer from a particular discomfort, but that he or she is fatefully connected to it. If one of the remedies is ineffective, another might be more suitable. It is not unusual that more than one remedy brings improvement. The collection of remedies has been passed on to me by my aunt, who, in turn, received them from her great-grandmother. These remedies have been passed down from ancient times, and I have used them successfully throughout my life. All are proven remedies from the Creator's great garden of nature. They will strengthen the self-healing process in all of us.

"First, there must be harmony between body and soul—that means inner tranquility between our thinking, our feeling, and our will. It makes no sense to look at health from a strictly mechanistic point of view. Twenty knee bends, half an hour of jogging, or six laps in the pool will not assure good health.

"To stay healthy, pay attention to your innate physical, intellectual, and psychological abilities. It's pointless to undertake an exercise routine just because it's fashionable. I'll try to show the general direction, but each person has to find for himself or herself what is appropriate or useful. One thing, however, is certain—fear will bring sickness. And fear is something that follows you *Payos* from cradle to grave.

"In this collection of recipes everybody will find the appropriate remedy for their particular weakness. The remedy will support the body's own immune system. In general, however, I recommend taking advantage of the power that resides in the almond. Eating three to six almonds a day will help us remain physically and mentally healthy well into old age.

"Our children, as soon as they can chew, eat two to three almonds daily as a life-giving support. Even our dog gets two almonds a day. He has been with us for 18 years. I bet you wouldn't have guessed that he's that old.

"Illness is a natural occurrence, like a volcanic eruption or a spring storm—the afflicted is forced to pause. The process of healing may be compared to swimming in the ocean. If you want to survive, swim with the tide, not against it."

Swimming against the tide, this wise healer explains, is what we do when we try to suppress illness with synthetic medications rather than helping the body overcome it.

"Not long ago a woman with a large open sore on her lower leg came to me for help. Her physician treated the sore locally, trying to close the wound as quickly as possible. His efforts were in vain; the sore broke open almost as soon as it seemed healed. I suggested keeping the sore open because her body was trying to expel toxins, a process not to be interfered with. To support this process, I applied leaves from the bear's breech (*Acanthus mollis*) plant for one week. At the end of a week the sore healed by itself.

"Even with minor discomfort, our whole organism is involved. It makes no sense, and it often is dangerous to treat only specific symptoms. Both our body and our soul need to be considered as a whole."

Fever is one way your body mobilizes its defenses, Pilar advises. Don't suppress this process. If necessary, use cold compresses on the lower legs. Use a cotton cloth, soaked in warm water, to which the juice of a lemon has been added. Wring out excess water, and wrap the cloth around the legs. Use another dry cotton cloth on top of the wet cloth, and pull a woolen sock over the entire leg. Avoid contact with cold air. For very high fever, repeat compresses every half hour.

Boil a twig of rosemary in water and keep a washcloth and a dry towel handy. Have all this in easy reach next to your bed. After an episode of heavy perspiration, wash yourself quickly to remove toxins from your skin. Then, dry yourself thoroughly. Change nightgown and bed linen. Don't reuse the linen and garment soaked with perspiration. Otherwise, the toxins your body has just gotten rid of will be reabsorbed through the skin.

Choose the young pale green shoots of nettle plants before they become sharp and bristly.

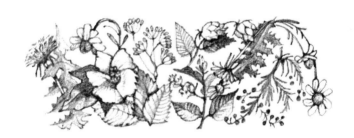

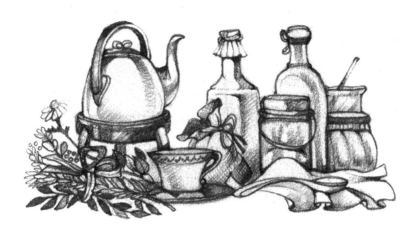

——— 3 ———
PILAR'S SECRET MEDICINE CHEST

"My first task, the one I like best, is to preserve health," Pilar says. "As somebody whose responsibility is healing, I must make teaching prevention my first priority. To be effective in not only regaining, but also in keeping, life's energies at their best is my task. Prevention ensures fitness and happiness well into old age.

"For preventive measures I recommend what I consider Elixirs of Life. The first is a tonic I call the Heal-Everything Tonic, the second is the tonic Gitano Bitter, and the third is Gypsy's Fountain-of-Youth Tonic.

"I consider these three tonics the foundation on which my medicine rests.

"Let's begin with this magic threesome. The first two tonics are as opposite as the sun and moon. Yet they complement each other, like these two planets, that profoundly influence human beings every day."

Before Bati Purí reveals the secrets of Gypsy medicine, she reminisces—her eyes gazing at the poplar trees on the banks of the Ebro River—about when her aunt, then very old, passed these secrets on to her.

"It was so many years ago when she entrusted me with these secrets. I was still a child at the time, but she, nevertheless, chose me as her successor. This was the same way that she was chosen to be healer and to guard the sacred knowledge our ancestors gathered on their long journeys around the world."

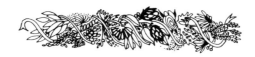

HEAL-EVERYTHING TONIC

2 handfuls mistletoe leaves   dry white wine
   with stems   genuine beeswax
7 mistletoe berries

Immediately after they are picked, crush 2 handfuls of European mistletoe leaves and stems by hand into small pieces and fill a dark brown bottle with them. Add 7 mistletoe berries, fill the bottle with dry, white wine, close the top with a natural cork, then seal the cork with real beeswax. The bottle with its contents is then buried one foot deep in the ground and left for 28 days. The top of the bottle must point toward the East. After one moon cycle the tonic will sufficiently mature.

Take one liqueur glass of the tonic twice daily, in the morning on an empty stomach and at night before retiring.

Caution: Mistletoe berries are poisonous; do not eat them.

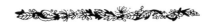

This tonic is assigned to the Sun. It gets its power from the mistletoe that grows on oak trees. About two thousand years ago, Druids, as white-clad priests of the Celtic tribes were called, worshipped this unusual evergreen plant with its pale berries. They considered them to possess magical powers. Harvesting the plant must be exactly timed to the night of the full moon that follows the winter solstice.

Pilar stresses the importance of harvesting mistletoe on that particular night since it is when the best energies are available to the plant. Also, the plant should not, under any circumstances, come in contact with any metal, except a golden sickle.

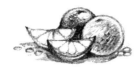

Pilar: "We consider this tonic a preventive. We take it even in the absence of any problems, because we know it strengthens the heart and the circulatory system. It also gently stimulates metabolism. If the blood pressure is too high, it helps lower it; if it is too low, it helps raise it. Heal-Everything Tonic activates the body's immune system."

Belief in the mistletoe plant's magical powers runs through European folklore. In Germany, for instance, it is known by various names—like witch bride, thunder broom, wood-of-the-cross, evergreen or wintergreen, bird's herb, and healing-all-ailments. In English it is sometimes called heal-all and devil's fugue.

Pilar is convinced that this tonic, taken in small doses, early enough and regularly, is effective against high blood pressure, strokes, heart attack, arteriosclerosis, rheumatism, gout, arthritis, and other ailments.

"I know," Pilar says, "that Heal-Everything Tonic increases the strength of body and mind, gives us courage and health, and helps us defend ourselves against diseases. I even think it can protect us against infections, tumors, and cancer."

21

GITANO BITTER

12 parts lovage root
15 parts angelica
5 parts tormentil
4 parts rhubarb
15 parts parsley
12 parts calamus
3 parts nutmeg
1.5 parts aloe vera
2.5 parts turmeric
10 parts gingerroot

1.3 parts galangal
1.2 parts crocus
15 parts masterwort
45 parts hawthorn
7 parts artichoke
14 parts yarrow
40 parts tea *de roca*
Spanish rockweed
100 proof alcohol

Grind the ingredients and steep them in alcohol. Let stand in the dark for 13 days, shaking the container once every day. On the 14th day, add rainwater equal to the amount of alcohol.

Take 1 liqueur glass twice daily after a meal.

This second life elixir is assigned to the Moon and the tides. Pilar considers its healing powers nothing short of magical. It stimulates digestion, strengthens the stomach and intestines, cleanses the blood, detoxifies and supports the pancreas. This tonic is an effective preventive and activates the body's immune system. It serves as a remedy to treat acute problems, like gastrointestinal cramps and colics.

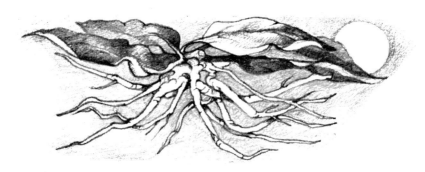

Gypsy Fountain of Youth

The Gypsy fountain of youth is wild garlic (*Allium ursinum*). This herb was well known to the Celts, Teutonic tribes, and ancient Romans. They gave this unassuming, wild plant of the lily family the name *herba salutaris*, "healing herb."

However, it has fallen into oblivion. But Gypsies gather and eat wild garlic every spring; that's probably why it is also known as Gypsy herb.

Ideally, wild garlic should be eaten fresh in the spring, before the plant starts to bloom. Add it to your diet for at least six weeks. Take a handful to eat with bread, add to salad, or mix with cottage cheese.

Wild garlic cleanses the blood and intestines. It improves the intestinal flora and is effective against acne, fungus, and eczema. It also lowers high blood pressure, fights arteriosclerosis, and increases the body's immune system. Also, Gypsies take wild garlic during epidemics for protection against infectious diseases.

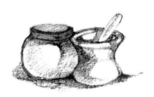

WILD GARLIC IN OLIVE OIL

To have wild garlic available during the year, the leaves are harvested just prior to blooming. Cut leaves into small pieces, put them in a dark bottle with a wide neck and add cold-pressed olive oil. Close the bottle and protect it from light.

Take one tablespoon daily.

If your supply runs out, regular garlic may be substituted. Simply use some garlic cloves and fill the container with oil as above. Prepare a tincture of wild garlic so that you can gain garlic's benefits when the fresh plant is not available.

GYPSY HERB TINCTURE

Harvest the leaves of the wild garlic plant just after dawn. To avoid losing the delicate, valuable essential oils, cut leaves immediately into small pieces. Pack leaves tightly into a container and seal tightly. Pour 180 proof alcohol over the leaves, making sure you cover them completely. Let them cure in a dark place for 28 days, shaking the container three times daily. On the 29th day, strain the contents through a gauze cloth and use a dropper to fill a dark bottle. Close the bottle tightly.

Take 20 drops three times daily just before a meal in water, tea, or directly on the tongue.

Pilar always has these three preparations, Heal-Everything Tonic, Gitano Bitter, and fountain-of-youth tonic made from wild garlic—Wild Garlic in Olive Oil or Gypsy Herb Tincture—in supply. They occupy a whole shelf in her trailer.

Pilar also keeps on hand thirteen other essential remedies—Golden Remedy for the Circulatory System, Rosemary–Sage–Red Wine Tonic, Whole Arnica Tincture, Soul-Refreshing Tonic, Banish Pain Tonic, Valerian Wine, Bride-of-the-Sun Salve, Saint-John's-Wort Oil, Blossom Oil, Thyme–Iodine Tonic, Coltsfoot Gargle, and Pilar's Cough Syrup. (Recipes for these remedies appear later in this book.)

ROSEMARY–SAGE–RED WINE TONIC

This tonic is used for recuperation from an illness.

Mix 1 handful each of rosemary and sage, and fill a stone jar. Add 1 litre of dry red wine; close the jar and let the contents rest for 13 hours. Heat the jar in a water bath for 30 minutes; do not let the water come to a boil. Let the jar cool to body temperature and add 3 tablespoons of honey. After one hour, strain the mixture through gauze, and fill a dark bottle that can be tightly closed.

Daily drink one liqueur glass before lunch and dinner.

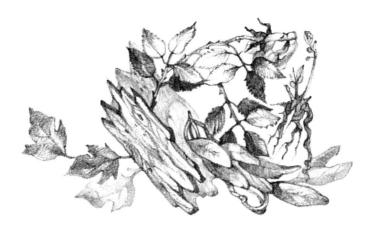

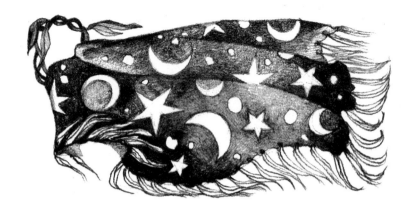

4

COLDS AND FLU

Gypsies, with their migratory way of life, are more exposed to the elements and solar radiation that those of us who live in solid houses. That has made them experts in treating colds, flus, hoarse throats, tonsillitis, bronchitis, sinus infections, and illnesses triggered by hypothermia. A sick person cannot travel, at least not comfortably.

I asked Pilar why the collection of remedies for colds and flu is so extensive.

"You should stop to look at the practical side of an application. Of course, we pay particular attention to infectious ailments triggered when a person gets cold, from prevention to cure."

"Is a cold a sign of a psychological ailment?"

"You are a typical Paya, always thinking of labels and categories. What is completely natural for every Gitano, you seem unable to understand. Everything that happens to us, including an illness, is predestined, fate. It's too bad, when you don't take an illness seriously; when you do not recognize it early enough and take precautions. In this sense, of course, a cold knocks at the door, the outer shell of your body, and asks to be let in. You must allow this uninvited guest to come in whether you want to or not. You can learn from its arrival if you are open and if you do not treat the guest with disdain. If you treat this uninvited guest well, he may turn around, politely say good-bye, and not come in at all.

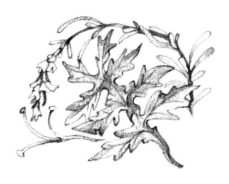

"We believe that every illness, even an insignificant one, is an important event in your life. If you know how to handle it, it will make you stronger. However, it also could weaken you and lead to serious or chronic diseases. In any case, you must learn to read the sign that an ailment gives you.

"If someone comes down with one of the many symptoms of a cold, don't look simply for a runny nose or sore throat. Symptoms are a sign of a general ailment. We see the different symptoms of a cold and realize they are part of a whole. We must give the organism of the sick person the support needed to fight the infection effectively from inside."

The Gypsy healer warns us not to suppress cold symptoms with synthetically produced pills—hoping for a quick fix.

"We must try to cure a cold from the inside. Otherwise, we may be faced, sometimes many years later, when the original infection has been forgotten, with disastrous consequences. The body takes revenge when it is not given the chance to gather the necessary strength to overcome an illness—when it has merely been repaired like a broken machine.''

Since Gypsies understand that the human organism is a whole system, they are careful not to take a cold lightly. They make sure that even such a seemingly trivial illness is well treated and properly cured. When the first symptoms of a cold appear, like sore throat, itchy nose, sneezing, chills, shivering, or cold feet, Pilar has a patent remedy at hand, Thyme–Iodine Tonic.

However, when someone is unable to get rid of the "uninvited guest at the door," Pilar prescribes absolute bed rest.

"I know it is a nuisance and boring," says Pilar. "But only in bed, where warmth supports perspiration, can a cold be treated successfully. Sometimes it might only take six to eight hours.

"We say, 'A cold takes three days in coming, three days staying, and three days leaving,' " I told Pilar.

Pilar smiles. "You can get rid of a cold much faster than that."

Pilar wraps her patients from head to toe in a so-called Spanish coat. The wrap, made from pure linen, aids perspiration, which opens the pores and helps the body rid itself of illness-causing germs. Pilar also gives the patient Anise–Willow Bark Tea. For the same symptoms, Pilar has a second, very effective remedy, Orrisroot–Lungwort Tea. Both are excellent sudorific teas.

Pilar's secret aid is Acid Air, which soothes irritated tissues and bronchial tubes. It supports Pilar's other remedies and makes breathing easier. This is important where air is dry or air-conditioned, both of which Pilar considers unhealthy.

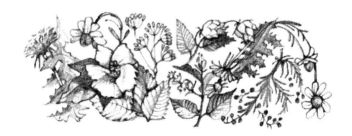

ACID AIR

For Acid Air, mix apple or wine vinegar with water at a ratio of one to two (say, 1 cup vinegar and 2 cups water). Bring the mixture to a boil, preferably in an earthenware pot, then place it on a trivet, and let it evaporate in the bedroom.

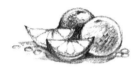

We all know by now how effective vitamin C is in preventing and fighting off a cold or flu. Pilar, however, suggests using natural vitamin C from a lemon, orange, or pomegranate. She is convinced that only natural plants can give us the strength to get well.

Pilar further suggests that the patient fast to gain energy, usually used for digestion, to fight the infection.

"Fast for at least three days. Drink plenty of fresh orange juice, if available, or any other freshly squeezed or pressed fruit juice. Carrot juice is a must! Drink lots of liquids to flush out toxins through the kidneys."

To increase kidney activity, Pilar recommends a mild Dog Rose–Chamomile Tea.

To generate new energy, Pilar recommends Heal-Everything Tonic.

"Don't forget that an illness, like a cold, may take a different course for different people. However, it always takes the route through a patient's weak spots. While one person easily gets bronchitis, another person's cold will settle into the sinuses, causing an infection. That's why one remedy is more effective for one person than for another. So, I sometimes give different recommendations for treating the same symptoms. When patients listen to their inner voice, they will be able to determine which remedies are best. Sometimes it is good to switch between remedies (teas, liniments, inhalations), because this will stimulate the body's immune system."

Bronchial Asthma

PILAR'S CHEST TEA

lungwort
mallow blossoms
lavender blossoms
coltsfoot leaves

Mix 1 handful each of lungwort, mallow blossoms, lavender blossoms, and coltsfoot leaves. Use 1 tablespoon of the mixture for every cup of boiling water. Let steep for 13 minutes.

Drink 1 cup three to four times a day. If desired, the tea may be sweetened with honey. "At the onset of an episode of bronchial asthma, rub the upper body and the back vigorously, until the skin is red. Try to calm the patient with gentle words and, if possible, with soothing music. Reduce fear!"

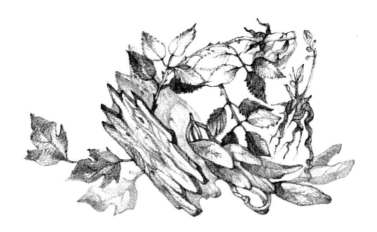

Bronchitis

PINE RESIN MILK

Dissolve 1 teaspoon of pine resin, 1 drop of lavender oil, and 1 spoonful of honey in 1 cup of warm milk.

Drink one cup three times daily. This remedy is also very effective for bronchial asthma accompanied by cough.

TEA FOR A COUGH

thyme

eucalyptus leaves

sage

black elderberry blossoms

Mix 1 handful each of thyme and eucalyptus leaves and one-half handful sage and black elderberry blossoms. Steep ingredients in boiling water for 13 minutes.

Drink one cup three to six times daily. Prepare enough tea to last for a day; keep the unused portion in a thermos bottle. Again, this remedy may be helpful for bronchial asthma accompanied by a cough.

ORRISROOT–ENGLISH IVY TINCTURE

Gather 1 handful orrisroot and 2 handfuls ivy (*Hedera helix*) leaves. Cut the orrisroot and ivy leaves into small pieces. Fill a bottle with them and add 150 proof alcohol. Let the mixture steep in the sun for 28 days; shake the bottle well once a day. Pour the contents through a strainer, and fill bottles with a dropper.

Add 10 drops of the tincture to a spoonful of brown sugar. Increase the number of drops as necessary. This remedy is also good for coughs.

ONION MILK

onions
clove
brown sugar
thyme twig
milk

Slice 3 large onions, discarding only the very outer skin, and layer them in a pot. Add 1 clove, 1 teaspoon of brown sugar, and 1 twig of thyme. Cover the ingredients with water and simmer at least 2 hours. Strain the contents through a gauze cloth; then squeeze out onion juice in a cheesecloth. Prior to application, add ½ cup of onion juice to ½ cup of hot milk.

Drink 2 to 3 cups daily. This is also very effective for bronchial asthma accompanied by coughing.

Pilar adds: "A gentle massage often brings relief, diminishing coughing spells. I massage throat, neck, and shoulders, and move my hands gently across the skin and muscles between the ribs."

Colds and Chills

THYME–IODINE TONIC

Use 1 tablespoon of thyme per cup of water. Pour boiling water over the thyme. Steep for 13 minutes. Let cool to lukewarm, and add 2 drops of iodine.

This Thyme–Iodine Tonic should be taken only once. (Do not use the principle "More is better." It can have the opposite effect.)

Caution: People with hyperthyroidism should not take this remedy.

"This is truly a magical tonic; it contains the power of the ocean. It sets in motion a kind of 'wave' within the body that may stop infectious germs in their tracks. But if you delay taking the remedy for just an hour—perhaps you want to do some shopping or you can't leave work—you'll miss the critical point." The Bati Purí adds, "Because, in all things, timing must be right.

"In the past, when iodine was not readily available in stores, my teacher, my aunt, used seaweed from the ocean—either fresh or dried."

ANISE–WILLOW BARK TEA

anise
linden blossoms
black elderberry blossoms
rosemary
ground willow bark

Mix 1 handful each of anise, linden blossoms, black elderberry blossoms, and rosemary with 1 tablespoon ground willow bark. Use 1 tablespoon per cup of tea. Cover mixture with boiling water. Steep for 15 minutes.

Sip one cup of tea two to three times a day.

This remedy is a good sudorific (it makes you sweat). Therefore, the patient must remain in bed. After sweating has subsided, quickly rub the patient with a sponge dipped in cold water, then wrap him or her in a previously warmed towel.

ORRISROOT–LUNGWORT TEA

orrisroot
wormwood leaves
chamomile blossoms
lungwort
ground willow bark

Mix 1 handful each of orrisroot, wormwood leaves, chamomile blossoms, and lungwort with 1 tablespoon of ground willow bark. Use 1 tablespoon for each cup of tea. Cover with boiling water and steep for 13 minutes.

Sip the tea, as hot as possible. Sweeten with honey if desired. This tea is also a sudorific.

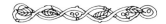

DOG ROSE–CHAMOMILE TEA

dog rose hips
chamomile blossoms
juniper berries
Italian parsley root

Gather 1 handful each of dog rose hips, chamomile blossoms, and juniper berries with ¼ handful of Italian parsley root. Mix ground dog rose hips with the parsley root, and cut into small pieces. Add the blossoms and berries. For one cup of tea, cover 1 tablespoon of the mixture with boiling water. Steep for 13 minutes.

Drink 1 to 3 cups of tea daily. This tea stimulates the kidneys.

Sore Throat and Hoarseness

LEMON–SALT GARGLE

Mix the juice of a lemon with 1 pinch of sea salt. Add 1 teaspoon of the mixture to a glass of water.

Three to four times a day gargle with the lemon–salt water.

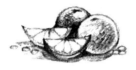

HONEY CANDY

Chew on a thumb-size piece of honeycomb as long as possible. Discard leftover wax from the comb.

Use the last two remedies, Lemon–Salt Gargle and Honey Candy, together. Both are very effective for hoarseness, tonsillitis, and pharyngitis.

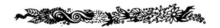

COLTSFOOT GARGLE

coltsfoot blossoms and leaves
English oak bark

Grind up ½ handful of English oak bark with wooden mortar and pestle. Cover with 1 quart of water. Let steep overnight. Add ½ handful each of coltsfoot leaves and coltsfoot blossoms, and warm slowly over a low flame. Remove from heat just before the mixture boils. Steep for 13 minutes. Strain through a gauze cloth.

Gargle with the liquid several times a day. It helps relieve tonsillitis.

QUINCE WINE

2 ripe quinces	2 cloves
1 rosemary twig	1 litre dry white wine
1 thyme twig	2 tablespoons honey

Wash and cut up quinces. Add rosemary, thyme, and cloves. Put ingredients in a container. Bring dry white wine to a boil, and add to the herb mixture. Let cool. When cool, cover the container securely with a linen cloth and a wooden lid. Let cure for 28 days. Then filter through a gauze cloth, add honey, and pour the wine into dark bottles.

For sore throat, hoarseness, tonsillitis, and pharyngitis, take 1 tablespoon three times daily.

Cough

PILAR'S COUGH SYRUP

Mix ½ cup each of pine resin and cold-pressed olive oil to a creamy consistency. Add 7 drops of thyme oil.

Smooth the salve onto the chest and back, cover with cotton padding, and wrap the upper body in a woolen cloth.

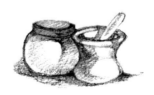

COLTSFOOT SYRUP

coltsfoot
ground willow bark
honey
dry white wine

Pick coltsfoot at noon one day before a new moon. Wash colts-foot leaves, blossoms, and stems. Dry well and put 10 handfuls of coltsfoot into an earthenware pot. Grind willow bark with a wooden mortar and pestle and sprinkle 2 tablespoons of ground willow on coltsfoot. Add 1 cup of honey to 1 litre of dry white wine, then add to the coltsfoot mixture. Press coltsfoot down in the container, and weigh it down with a stone so that it is well covered by the wine. Add more wine if needed.

Carefully cover the pot with a linen cloth, then a wooden lid. Bury the pot in the ground, and cover it with at least 8 inches of earth. After 28 days, unearth the pot. Bring the mixture to a boil and strain through a gauze cloth. Bring the liquid to a boil again until it has a syrupy consistency. Fill green or brown glass containers with the syrup. Seal containers tightly.

Take 1 teaspoon three times a day. The dose may be increased as necessary. This syrup is also effective for bronchial catarrh and smoker's cough.

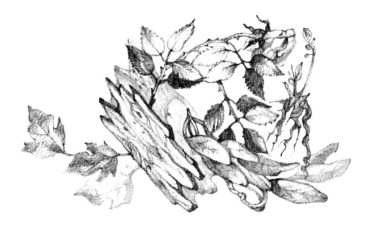

EUCALYPTUS FACIAL STEAM

Grind 1 handful of cypress fruits with a wooden mortar and pestle. Cut up 1 handful of eucalyptus leaves, and mix with cypress fruit. Add 2 quarts of cold water. Bring mixture to a boil and simmer for 5 minutes. Strain.

Then hold your face over the steam and inhale deeply. Cover your head with a towel so that the steam does not escape. This is also a good remedy for hoarseness and pharyngitis.

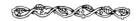

Sinus Infections

THYME STEAM

Make a thyme tea with 1 handful thyme; let boil for 3 minutes. Remove from the flame, strain, and add 5 drops of bergamot oil.

With a towel covering your head, inhale the steam. This remedy is also recommended for bronchial infections.

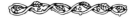

Laryngitis

CHAMOMILE GARGLE

Make chamomile tea with 1 tablespoon of chamomile blossoms per cup. Add 2 teaspoons of sea salt to every cup of tea.

Gargle three to four times daily.

LEMON OIL

Crush 2 garlic cloves in a small bowl, add 2 tablespoons of olive oil, and mix well. Add juice of one lemon to the oil in small drops, as though you were making mayonnaise.

Take 1 teaspoon three times a day.

"I recommend this Lemon Oil remedy for illnesses that affect the voice, like laryngitis, pharyngitis, and vocal cord infections. This remedy has been well tested by our people who use their voices with gusto—laughing, singing, talking."

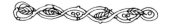

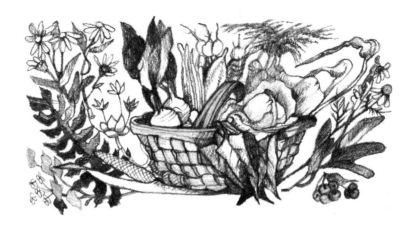

5

HEART AND CIRCULATORY SYSTEM

"You and your heart belong together like the Moon and the Sun, like the wind and the ocean," says Pilar. "Everything you experience, everything you take in, good and bad, leaves its mark on your heart. And your heart 'shapes' you."

Arteriosclerosis

FRUIT VINEGAR–HONEY DRINK

Mix well 1 tablespoon each of fruit vinegar (such as apple vinegar) and honey in 1 cup of water.

Slowly sip this drink in the morning. It works best when taken regularly.

"This Fruit Vinegar–Honey Drink is also an excellent preventive remedy. It rids blood vessels of deposits and keeps them young and pliable. The old saying, 'A person is only as strong as his vessel' is true."

In addition, Pilar suggests that people with arteriosclerosis use only olive oil and eat lots of onions, spinach, nettle salad, Gypsy's herb (wild garlic), dandelion, sorrel, and watercress—always fresh. Also eat six almonds and 1¾ ounces of fresh yeast each day. Eat only coarse whole wheat or rye bread. No pork!

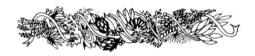

MISTLETOE–FENNEL TEA

mistletoe
kidney bean pods
mallow blossoms
fennel seeds
yarrow

Gather 1 handful each of European mistletoe, kidney bean pods, mallow blossoms, fennel seeds, and yarrow. Cut mistletoe, bean pods, and yarrow into small pieces. Mix with the mallow blossoms and fennel seeds. Use 1 tablespoon for each cup of tea. Cover the mixture with boiling water; let steep in a covered pan for 13 minutes. Strain through a gauze cloth.

Drink a cup of warm tea three times a day. Sweeten with honey, if you wish.

High Blood Pressure

HONEY–RICE DIET

8 ounces brown rice	3½ ounces honey
1½ pounds fruit or fresh fruit juices	⅓ ounce fresh yeast

Steam rice until done. Do not add salt. Mix the 1½ pounds fruit or fruit juice with the rice. When cool, add the 3½ ounces honey. To avoid loss of nutrients, the honey should not be heated above 105° F.

Divide the mixture into seven portions. In the morning, on an empty stomach, eat ⅙ ounce of fresh yeast followed by the first portion of the honey rice with fruit. At night, before retiring, eat the other ⅙ ounce yeast followed by the last portion of rice. Eat the other five rice portions spaced throughout the day.

Drink nothing after the last meal, except Heal-Everything Tonic.

Pilar: "In addition, I strongly recommend remaining calm. *Fear* of high blood pressure by itself can increase blood pressure. Measure blood pressure only in the morning, immediately after waking up, when you're relaxed."

VALERIAN–BITTER ORANGE TEA

valerian root
lavender blossoms
rosemary
bitter orange leaves
chamomile blossoms

Cut into small pieces 1 handful of valerian root; crush 1 handful of bitter orange leaves in your hands. Mix with ½ handful of rosemary, ½ handful of lavender blossoms, and 1 handful of chamomile blossoms.

Use 1 tablespoon of the valerian–bitter orange mixture for each cup of tea. Pour boiling water over the herb mixture. Steep in a covered pot for 13 minutes.

Drink 1 cup of lukewarm tea twice daily; sweeten with honey.

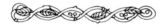

OLIVE LEAF TEA

olive leaves
garlic cloves

Pour 1 quart of boiling water over 1 handful of olive leaves. Steep in a covered pot for 13 minutes. Strain through gauze, and add the juice from 7 garlic cloves.

For 1 week, sip a cup of tea twice a day, morning and evening. Then stop for a week. Repeat the procedure for another week. If necessary, continue treatment this way, in alternating weeks.

Nervous Heart Condition

VALERIAN–RASPBERRY TEA

raspberry leaves
valerian root
bitter orange leaves
wormwood
balm

Cut up 1 handful of valerian root. Crush 1 handful each of raspberry leaves, bitter orange leaves, and balm and ½ handful of wormwood (absinthe) in your hands. Use 1 tablespoon of this mixture per cup of tea. Pour boiling water over the dry mixture. Steep, covered, for 13 minutes.

Drink 1 cup of warm tea morning and night. The tea may be sweetened with honey.

Varicose Veins

COMFREY–CYPRESS SALVE

1 handful comfrey roots
1 handful cypress fruit

1 handful goat butter (or neutral base)

Comfrey roots are gathered in the spring or the fall, then well scrubbed and quickly dried in the sun. They should be stored in a tightly covered container.

Grind 1 handful of comfrey with mortar and pestle. Remove the marrow of 1 handful cypress fruits and grind with mortar and pestle. Mix equal parts of comfrey and cypress fruit marrow. Melt 1 handful of goat butter over low heat (don't overheat), add the pulverized mixture, and stir for 15 minutes. Strain the mixture. Fill an earthenware or dark glass container with the salve. Protect the container from light; keep it in a cool place. (A neutral base, available in pharmacies, may be substituted for goat butter.)

Apply to affected veins three to four times a day.

High or Low Blood Pressure

GOLDEN REMEDY FOR THE CIRCULATORY SYSTEM

1 handful European
   mistletoe leaves
1 tablespoon periwinkle

1 tablespoon olive leaves
1 teaspoon nettle juice

Crush and mix 1 handful of European mistletoe leaves and 1 tablespoon each of periwinkle and olive leaves in your hands. Put the leaves in an earthenware pot, cover with 1 quart of cold rainwater. Let steep, covered, overnight or for 13 hours. Strain through a gauze cloth.

Add 1 teaspoon of nettle juice just before drinking. Prepare nettle juice by crushing the leaves with a mortar and pestle; then press them through a gauze cloth.

Drink 1 cup three times daily, sweetened with honey if you wish.

Due to its balancing effects, this remedy is helpful for both high and low blood pressure. Also try Dandelion–Mistletoe Coffee and Valerian Wine.

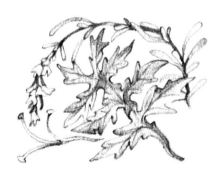

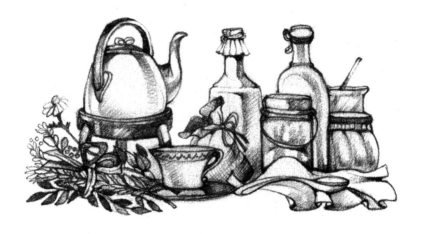

---6---

DIGESTIVE SYSTEM

"Our well-being and our digestive system are connected like Siamese twins. That's why I can't understand why one would try to heal gallbladder colic and a stomach ulcer separately, as though they were disconnected from the human being afflicted," Pilar says.

She gets up, bends down to pick up a pebble, and flings it into the river. "We usually get stomachaches when we feel over-extended, or the opposite, when we are not challenged enough—when we cannot fulfill our ambitions."

"What do you suggest for someone with such a problem?" I ask.

"Of course, the person could try my remedies. They will help alleviate symptoms. But the person's inner struggle must also be faced. "For instance, if there's a lot of pressure at work, one may literally feel pain in the stomach just thinking of the boss or colleagues. If you have to work, you can't just take off and quit. You must bravely endure the people around you. Arm yourself with mental calluses. Endure it like bad weather, something all of us, especially we Gypsies, cannot escape either."

For people who find themselves in such a dilemma, Pilar suggests they find a place and time where they can be themselves—run free.

"We all know what gives us joy. There is no rule of thumb. Some of us like classical music, others like dancing at the disco, and still others would prefer watching soccer. Every one of us has a weak point in his constitution. Find yours, then tailor your approach to a problem accordingly.

"The Sun of our digestive system is the liver. Language suggests how close the liver is to the source of life—liver = live. Language can guide us to the source of life. Avoid toxins for just one month and the liver will be as good as new.

"Since I know people, and since Gypsies are also guilty of indulging in a bit of the 'good life,' I have a whole collection of recipes that are helpful for stimulating our digestive system and staying healthy."

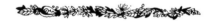

Appetizer

BITTER ORANGE SYRUP

bitter oranges
white wine
brown sugar

Wash 3 organically grown bitter oranges. Peel the skin as thin as possible so that most of the white portion remains on the fruit. Cut the skin into small pieces and cover with 1 litre of white wine. Let boil for 13 minutes, preferably in a copper pot.

Peel the white portion of the skin of the fruit. Cut up the fruit and add to the wine mixture. Add 13 seeds from the fruit and stir in 13 tablespoons of brown sugar. Let boil for 30 minutes, stirring frequently. Remove the seeds, and pour the syrup into glass jars that can be tightly covered.

Take 1 tablespoon in the morning and at night. Children are fond of this appetizer. Bitter orange syrup is also a mild laxative.

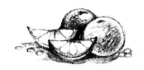

Lack of Appetite

MISTLETOE WINE

centaury root
mistletoe leaves
red wine
juniper berries

Cut 1 handful of European centaury root into small pieces, and mix with 1 handful of European mistletoe leaves. Pour 1 litre of red wine over the plants, and cover with a lid. Steep overnight. The next morning, bring to a boil and simmer 10 minutes.

Grind 3 juniper berries with mortar and pestle, and add to the mixture. Let simmer 3 more minutes. Add 1 tablespoon of flowering lemon balm. Remove the pot from the fire, cover, and allow the mixture to cool. Strain through a gauze cloth and fill bottles that can be tightly closed.

Drink 1 liqueur glass of Mistletoe Wine twice daily before a meal.The wine is an excellent appetite stimulant and a good remedy for anorexia.

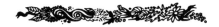

For Weight Loss

Appetite Suppressants

BRAN BREAKFAST

fragrant valerian root
1 handful wheat bran

1 tablespoon dog rose hips
1 teaspoon honey

Harvest fragrant valerian root in the spring or fall (not summer). Clean well with a root brush, and let it air dry in the shade. Store it in a linen sack in a place where air can circulate. When needed, cut enough root into small pieces to make 1 heaping tablespoon. Cover with water. Steep, covered, overnight. Warm the liquid to body temperature, and strain through a gauze cloth.

Soak 1 handful of wheat bran in this liquid, and add 1 tablespoon of dog rose hips (*or* 1 teaspoon of dog rose hips and 1 teaspoon of honey).

Eat in the morning on an empty stomach. This appetite suppressant is a proven Gypsy recipe for losing weight.

BLOOD-CLEANSING TEA

dandelion root
artichoke leaves

Grind up half of a dandelion root (the size of your thumb) to make dandelion root powder. Cut up a few artichoke leaves. Mix 1 heaping teaspoon of dandelion root powder and ½ teaspoon of artichoke leaves. Cover with boiling water. Let steep in a covered pot for 13 minutes, and strain through gauze.

Sip 2 to 3 cups of this tea, not too hot, daily. A little honey may be added if you find this too bitter. Drink this tea with Bran Breakfast to stimulate the liver and gallbladder.

Purification
PILAR'S WEIGHT LOSS TEA

1 handful hibiscus blossoms
1 handful fennel seeds
½ handful peppermint leaves
3 tablespoons rosemary
3 tablespoons lady's mantle (dewcup)
4 tablespoons yarrow
4 tablespoons melilot
1 tablespoon lemon balm
2 tablespoons birch leaves
2 tablespoons nettle leaves
2 tablespoons horsetail
1 tablespoon hops
1 tablespoon dandelion leaves and blossoms
1 tablespoon wormwood (absinthe)
1 teaspoon chamomile
1 teaspoon restharrow
1 tablespoon linden blossoms
2 teaspoons fumitory
1 tablespoon black mulberry leaves
2 teaspoons sandalwood

Mix these ingredients and use 1 tablespoon for each cup of tea. Pour the dry tea into an earthenware or enamel pot, and add boiling water. Quickly bring to a boil, then remove from heat, and let steep, covered, for 5 minutes. Strain through a gauze cloth.

Sip the tea lukewarm; take 2 to 4 cups daily. Prepare enough tea for a day, and keep it in a thermos bottle.

Sweeten the tea with honey, brown sugar, or artificial sweetener if you wish. This tea will detoxify the system without causing hunger sensations.

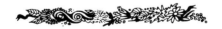

Other Digestive Ailments

Vomiting

PAPRIKA HONEY

Grind paprika with a mortar and pestle. Add 1 pinch of paprika from freshly ground sweet pepper to 1 teaspoon of honey.

Take 1 teaspoon three times a day to fight nausea.

Diarrhea

TANGY CHAMOMILE TEA

chamomile blossoms
whortleberries (blueberries)
English oak bark, pulverized

Mix 1 handful of German chamomile blossoms with 25 dried whortleberries (blueberries) and 1 tablespoon of pulverized English oak bark. Use 1 tablespoon for each cup of water. Cover with cold water, then bring to a boil, and let boil for 3 minutes. Remove from fire, cover, steep for 13 minutes. Strain through gauze.

Drink 1 cup of the tea—not too hot—three times a day. This tea is also effective for nausea and vomiting.

Gallbladder Infection

WILD DAISY TEA

nettle leaves

horehound

English daisy blossoms

Pour 1 litre of vigorously boiling water over 1 handful each of nettle leaves and English daisy blossoms and ½ handful of horehound. Steep in a covered pot for 10 minutes. Strain the tea through gauze.

Drink 1 cup of tea every 2 hours throughout the day. This tea is also recommended for liver disorders.

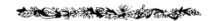

Gallstones

OLIVE OIL–LEMON JUICE CURE

olive oil

lemon juice

sea water

Mix 1 tablespoon of olive oil with 1 teaspoon of lemon juice, adding the oil one drop at the time to the juice. Heat 1 cup of sea water.

Day 1—Take 1 tablespoon of olive oil and 1 teaspoon of lemon juice. Drink 1 cup of sea water. Then lie on your right side for half an hour. Relax. Visualize the mineral deposits or stones in your gallbladder being dissolved.

Day 2—Repeat the procedure for day 1 here and for the days that follow, but increase the olive oil to 2 tablespoons. Continue to use just 1 teaspoon of lemon juice for all 6 days. Day 3— Increase olive oil to 3 tablespoons, Day 4—to 4 tablespoons, Day 5—5 tablespoons, and Day 6—6 tablespoons.

Gastritis

COMFREY POWDER

The root of the comfrey plant should be harvested during the first night of the new moon after the summer solstice. (Remember not to take out the root in its entirety. Leave the strongest portion in the earth to guarantee survival of the plant.) Scrub the root well and immediately hang it up to dry in direct sunlight. Usually avoid exposure to direct sunlight when drying herbs; in this case, sunlight prevents the plant materials with high water content from becoming moldy. Store the root in a linen sack.

When needed, pulverize a piece of root, and take 1 pinch directly on your tongue. Accumulate saliva before swallowing the powder.

Comfrey powder is recommended for heartburn and other gastrointestinal illnesses.

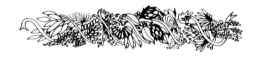

Liver Detoxification

ARTICHOKE DRINK

1 handful artichoke leaves	1 litre dry red wine
1 handful rosemary	13 saffron stigmas

Cut artichoke leaves and rosemary into small pieces at night during a full moon. Mix both and pour red wine over them. Add saffron stigmas. Pour the mixture into a bottle, close tightly, and bury the bottle in the earth. Let it rest until the next new moon. Then unearth the bottle and strain the contents through gauze. Store the artichoke drink in a dark bottle.

Drink 1 liqueur glass in small sips twice a day after main meals. This drink is helpful for reducing the blood cholesterol level.

Hemorrhoids

CYPRESS PULP SALVE

1 handful cypress fruit pulp

1 handful yarrow blossoms

1 handful goat butter

Remove and grind the pulp from the cypress fruit with mortar and pestle. Crush yarrow blossoms. Melt goat butter over low heat, being careful the butter doesn't turn brown. Mix goat butter with the cypress pulp. Let the mixture cool, and place it in a dark place for three days.

After the third day, warm the mixture again over low heat. Strain through gauze and store. Use a container that can be tightly closed in a cool place.

Use the salve several times a day. Add a small amount to a piece of gauze and apply directly to the anus, particularly overnight. If necessary, insert some salve into the rectum.

To increase the shelf life of the salve, substitute a neutral salve base for the goat butter.

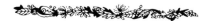

Stomach Disorders (Lack of Acidity)

VALERIAN–LEMON BALM TEA

1 handful valerian roots

½ handful green, unripened juniper berries

½ handful juniper bark

½ handful artichoke leaves

1 handful fennel seeds

1 handful lemon balm

Cut valerian roots and juniper bark into small pieces. Crush artichoke leaves in your hand. Lightly crush juniper berries (green, unripened). Mix ingredients with fennel seeds and lemon balm. Use 1 tablespoon per cup of water. Pour over boiling water mixture. Steep in a covered pot for 13 minutes. Strain through a gauze cloth.

Drink 1 cup of the tea, lukewarm, three times a day.

Stomach and Small Intestine Ulcers

ALMOND MILK

8 ounces sweet almonds
1 bitter almond
3 drops rosewater

½ lemon
1 quart rain or distilled water

Cover sweet almonds and bitter almond with boiling water. Steep 3 minutes, strain, and remove the brown skin. Dry peeled almonds in a cloth or towel. Grind almonds in a nut grinder. To make a paste, work the ground almonds with mortar and pestle, adding 2 to 3 tablespoons of rain or distilled water. Then add the remaining water, rosewater, and the juice of half a lemon. Let the mixture rest for 3 hours in a cool place. Strain the mixture through a gauze cloth. Pour into clean bottles and keep in the refrigerator. Almond milk prepared in such a way will stay fresh for 24 hours.

Divide the contents into three equal portions, and drink one in the morning, at noon, and at night.

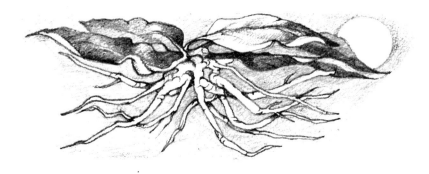

Heartburn

STOMACH WELLNESS TEA

catkins from hazelnut bush
chamomile blossoms
coltsfoot leaves

Cut ¼ cup of coltsfoot leaves into small pieces. Mix with 1 cup of hazelnut catkins and ½ cup of chamomile blossoms. Use 1 tablespoon for each cup of water. Pour boiling water over the dry tea. Cover and steep 15 minutes. Strain through a gauze cloth (not a metal strainer).

Drink one cup of tea that's not too hot after each meal. Do not sweeten the tea.

The mucilaginous substance contained in the Stomach Wellness Tea will coat the sensitive lining of the stomach with a protective film, which will shield the lining from irritating substances contained in food and drinks such as alcohol.

OAK BARK–ROSE TEA

English oak bark
rose leaves
long-spurred pansy roots
sage leaves
blackberry (brambleberry) leaves

Cut 1 handful each of English oak bark and long-spurred pansy roots into small pieces. Crush 1 handful of rose leaves, 1 handful of sage leaves, and ½ handful of blackberry leaves in your hand. Mix them well. Use 1 cup of water for each tablespoon of the dry tea mixture. Pour boiling water over the desired amount of tea. Cover and steep 13 minutes. Strain through gauze cloth.

Drink one cup of cold tea in small sips, three times a day.

Indigestion

CAROB–FIG BALLS

carob fruits

dried figs

orange oil

Crush 7 carob fruits (fenugreek may be substituted) with a wooden mortar and pestle. Cut 2 handfuls of dried figs into small pieces. Mix both fruits and add 3 drops of orange oil. If the mixture is too stiff, add a few drops of Gitano Bitter (see recipe on page 22). Form the dough into small balls.

Eat one ball, 3 times a day. Chew slowly, using lots of saliva. When the digestive problem is reduced, eat only twice a day, and eventually only once a day, until you have become regular. This remedy is also helpful for intestinal functions.

When in the desert, John the Baptist ate carob fruits, which he called wild honey.

Dried carob seeds were used in the Mediterranean and in East India as measuring weights by pharmacists, goldsmiths, and jewelers. One seed equaled 1 *carat*, the Arabic name of seeds of the carob tree. To this day, precious stones are measured in carats, with a metric weight of 200 milligrams.

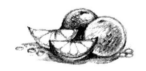

Hiccups

VALERIAN–RASPBERRY–SAGE TEA

1 handful valerian roots
1 handful blackberry
  (brambleberry) leaves
1 handful fennel seeds

1 handful chamomile
  blossoms
1 handful peppermint
  leaves
1 handful sage leaves

Cut valerian roots into small pieces. Crush blackberry (brambleberry) leaves and peppermint leaves in your hand. Mix both with chamomile blossoms and fennel seeds. Use 1 tablespoon for each cup of water. Cover mixture with boiling water. Steep in a covered pot for 13 minutes. Strain through gauze cloth.

Drink 1 cup of lukewarm tea three times a day.

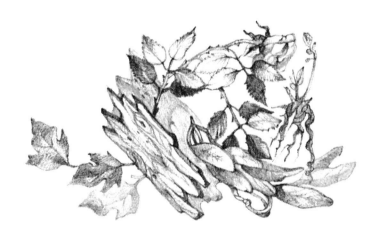

Intestinal Parasites

POMEGRANATE JUICE

Mix the juice of 1 ripe pomegranate and the juice of 2 garlic cloves. Add 1 to 2 teaspoons of honey and stir. You may increase the amount of honey, if you like.

Drink the juice before lunch for 13 days. Children, especially, enjoy this effective remedy.

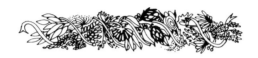

Constipation

PLUM JAM

4 pounds 6 ounces ripe plums	1 tablespoon apple vinegar
3½ ounces honey	3½ ounces tamarind jam

Put pitted plums and ⅓ of the pits into a large pot. Fill the pot with water and boil for one hour, uncovered. Stir occasionally and add more water if necessary. After an hour, remove the pits, and continue to let the mixture simmer for another 15 minutes. After the jam has cooled, add honey, apple vinegar, and tamarind jam. Pour the jam into glass containers that can be tightly sealed.

Take 1 tablespoon of plum jam in the morning on an empty stomach. Continue this treatment until you overcome constipation and under-activity of the intestines.

Chronic Constipation

HERBAL OIL

1 pint cold-pressed (extra virgin) olive oil
1 handful black elderberries
½ handful rosemary blossoms
1 tablespoon flax seeds
1 valerian root (½ thumb thickness)

Mix olive oil with rosemary blossoms and black elderberries. Shake well, and set aside in a dark place in a tightly sealed container for three days.

On the fourth day, crush flax seeds with mortar and pestle; add to the olive oil mixture. Crush valerian root and add to the oil. Shake the container vigorously. Seal tightly and set aside for 7 days, shaking the container twice a day, in the morning and at night. On the eighth day, strain the oil through a gauze cloth (do not use a metal strainer). Pour the oil into dark bottles and store in a dark place.

Take 1 tablespoon of the herbal oil in the morning on an empty stomach. If need be, take an additional tablespoon before the evening meal. This medicine also relieves the gallbladder and kills harmful intestinal bacteria. Take it until you regain regularity.

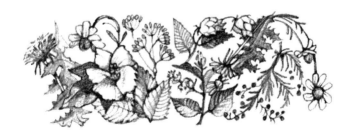

Stimulating Metabolism

PILAR'S SPRING CURE

Mix 1 handful each of watercress, dandelion, and blind nettle. Eat fresh as a salad for lunch and dinner with a dressing of olive or nut oil, vinegar, and sea salt. Make Spring Cure Salad the first course. When eaten regularly, this salad stimulates metabolism and is ideal for internal "spring housecleaning."

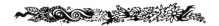

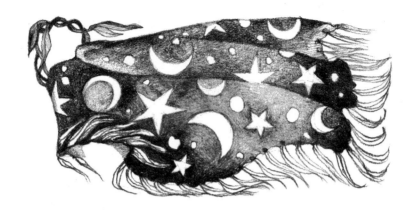

7

ELIMINATION ORGANS

"Before we talk about kidneys, I want to show you something," Pilar tells me, leading me out of the trailer park. Pilar stops in front of an olive tree, with a trunk about 40 inches around and leaves that glisten in the sun.

"This tree is more than a thousand years old," Pilar says, "may it live a thousand more." She reaches for a young branch that forks into two branches. She carefully strips the branch of its leaves and bark, which she puts in her big skirt pocket.

"You know what this is?"

She shows me the naked wood with a joint in the middle where it divides into a Y, like a butterfly's feeler. Both extensions are about the diameter of my little finger and half the length of my arm. I don't have a clue.

"It is a dowsing rod."

Pilar holds one end of the Y in her right hand and the other in her left with fingers closed over the wood. The stem of the

Y she points straight up to the sky. Pilar indicates that I should follow her. She goes forward, slowly, with her head slightly bowed. I count my steps as I follow—49 so far. Then, I notice the olive branch in Pilar's hands begin to shiver, first bending down toward the ground, then righting itself again, then rotating as if somebody wound it up.

"An underground water vein."

"How deep?" I ask.

"About 100 to 130 feet, perhaps. More measuring is necessary to get accurate information." Pilar steps aside, handing me the olive branch. "See if you can harness the rays of the earth and transfer them to another object."

I wonder whether Pilar is playing tricks with me. But the weight of the olive branch, at first so light, seems to grow heavier and heavier.

"Stop brooding," Pilar says. "Concentrate on the dowsing rod and what it wants to show you. Don't tense up."

I take three tentative steps, holding the olive branch upright. I feel, without any movement on my part, the branch beginning first to bend down, then righting itself again, followed by rotating movements that become faster and faster. My whole body vibrates.

"Enough," says Pilar, "come with me." She takes the dowsing rod out of my hand. Slowly we make our way back to the trailer camp. Before we reach Pilar's trailer, decorated with the sun, the moon, and stars, I feel a sharp pain in the lower portion of my back, on both sides of the spine. The pain begins to spread throughout my body. I grow pale; I tighten my jaws—it hurts so much.

"Yes, the kidneys," says Pilar. She looks at me encouragingly. "Don't worry, it will soon pass."

Pilar hands me a cup of tea. "You won't be harmed. I only wanted you to feel for yourself how dangerous it is to live on top of a water vein.

"Our kidneys are much influenced by water, the ocean, and the moon—all those energies in constant motion. That's why salt is so harmful for our kidneys, since it is part of the fossilized structure of minerals. Sea salt is much better. It contains all the many living and enriching components that are the source of life."

I ask what people prone to kidney problems and the organs connected with them should do to protect themselves.

"The first thing that comes to mind is the bad habit that all you 'sun-hungry' tourists have—sitting around in wet bathing suits! These people have no idea what harm they do to themselves!"

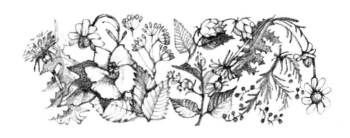

Bladder Infections

MISTLETOE–BLACK ELDERBERRY TEA

mistletoe leaves
birch leaves
black elderberry blossoms
bearberry leaves
chamomile blossoms

Crush 1 handful each of mistletoe plant and bearberry leaves in your hand. Mix with 1 handful each of black elderberry blossoms, bearberry leaves, and chamomile blossoms. Use 1 tablespoon for each cup of tea. Add the mixture to boiling water, and boil for 13 minutes more. Strain through a gauze cloth.

Drink 1 cup of lukewarm tea, three times a day, a half hour before a meal. Sip slowly. The tea may be sweetened with honey.

Kidney Complaints

COWSLIP–ELDERBERRY TEA

Add 3 quarts of cold water to 2 handfuls of nettle leaves and 1 handful each of black elderberries and cowslip blossoms in a large pot. Cover the pot and bring contents to a boil. Then, simmer for 3 minutes.

Slowly sip 1 cup of tea seven times a day. This tea also supports treatment of kidney infections and kidney stones.

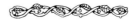

ELDERBERRY BARK TEA

Crush 1 handful of black elderberry bark with mortar and pestle. Put the crushed bark in an earthenware pot, and add one quart of cold water. Bring to a boil and simmer for 13 minutes. Strain through a gauze cloth.

Drink 4 to 5 cups of tea during the day. This tea has strong diuretic properties and aids treatment of kidney infections and kidney stones.

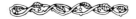

ROOT TEA

parsley roots
couch grass roots
rose blossoms

Cut 1 handful each of couch grass roots and parsley roots into small pieces. Add 2 quarts of water to the mixture. Bring to a boil in an earthenware pot; then simmer for 13 minutes. Remove from heat and stir in 1 handful of rose blossoms. Cover the pot and steep for 10 minutes. Strain through a gauze cloth.

Drink 5 to 7 cups of tea during the day. This tea is also recommended for the treatment of kidney infections and kidney stones.

Kidney Stones

ENGLISH OAK–SCOTCH BROOM TEA

acorns

Scotch broom blossoms and young twigs

wormwood

nettle roots

Grind 1 handful of acorns, and cut 1 handful of nettle roots into small pieces. Cut 1 handful of Scotch broom blossoms that have been picked before they have opened and young twigs with 1 handful of wormwood into small pieces. Mix all ingredients. Use 1 tablespoon for every cup of tea. Pour boiling water over the dry tea. Steep, covered, for 13 minutes. Strain through a gauze cloth.

Drink 1 cup of tea three times a day. The tea may be sweetened with honey.

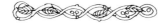

DOG ROSE HIPS–ROSEMARY TEA

2 handfuls dog rose hips
1 handful restharrow roots
1 handful basil
1 handful silver birch
  leaves

1 handful shelled kidney
  beans
½ handful rosemary

Cut restharrow roots into small pieces. Crush dog rose hips, silver birch leaves, and shelled kidney beans in your hands. Add basil and rosemary. Mix all ingredients. Use 1 teaspoon for each cup of tea. Let mixture boil for 7 minutes, preferably in an earthenware or enamel pot. Cover and steep for 13 minutes.

Sip 1 cup of hot tea three times a day for kidney infections. The tea may be sweetened with honey.

DANDELION–MISTLETOE COFFEE

Harvest dandelion roots in spring or fall. Air dry in the shade, never in the oven. Clean the roots well with a vegetable brush. Roast over low heat in an iron skillet until roots turn coffee brown. Let cool. Store in a tin canister or in a glass jar with a tightly sealed lid. Grind roots so they will be fresh when needed.

For each cup of coffee, use 1 teaspoon of the dandelion powder and 3 pinches of dried mistletoe leaves crushed with a mortar and pestle. To improve the taste, 1 teaspoon of real coffee may be added. Pour boiling water over the mixture, and steep for 6 minutes.

Sip 1 cup of the coffee three times a day. Do not use honey or sugar, since they diminish the healing effects of the bitter substances of the dandelion plant.

This remedy stimulates the heart and kidneys. It also helps regulate blood pressure—lowering high and elevating low blood pressure. It strengthens gastric juices, aids digestion, and helps the kidneys eliminate toxins from the body.

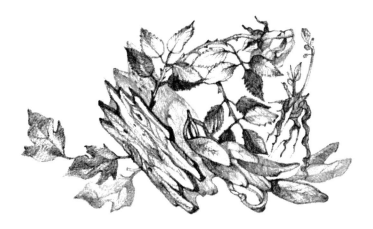

Kidney Stones

SEA FENNEL TEA

restharrow roots
valerian roots
bearberry leaves
sea fennel

Cut 1 handful each of restharrow roots and valerian roots into small pieces. Crush 1 handful each of sea fennel and bearberry leaves. Mix ingredients well. Use 1 tablespoon for each cup of tea. Pour boiling water over the mixture, and steep, covered, for 13 minutes. Strain through a gauze cloth.

Sip 1 cup of tea twice a day.

Pilar also recommends a sea-water cure for kidney stones. "The ocean's powerful healing energies will wash out the kidneys and dissolve the stones."

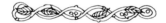

Prostate Problems

WILLOW-HERB TEA

Every man ought to know about this remedy. It works like magic. Gypsy men drink this tea as a preventive at the first sign of gray hair. For preventive measures, however, take only in small quantities, no more than a liqueur glass of tea daily.

For the tea use either of the willow-herbs *Epilobium roseum*, a small-leaved species, or *Epilobium montana*. Pick only those herbs that grow under or near an English oak tree.

Pick the leaves, blossoms, and twigs just after noon, when the sun is at its peak. Sun allows the essential oil of the plant to be at its best.

Dry and store the plant in a tightly covered jar. Crush leaves, blossoms, and twigs just before brewing the tea. Use 1 heaping tablespoon for each cup of tea. Pour boiling water over the dry tea, and steep for 10 minutes. Add 7 drops of Nettle Tincture (see below).

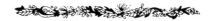

NETTLE TINCTURE

nettle roots
100 proof alcohol, not denatured

Clean and dry fresh nettle roots, and cut them into small pieces. Fill an earthenware or glass jar with the nettle roots. Tightly seal the container and put it in a warm place or in the sun for three days. Cover the roots with 100 proof alcohol and rain-water in a one-to-one ratio. Let it sit for one moon cycle (28 days), shaking the container every morning and evening. After 28 days strain the tincture through a gauze cloth, and fill bottles that can be tightly sealed.

Drink 1 cup of tea and 7 drops of nettle tincture in the morning and evening. As a preventive, drink just one liqueur glass of tea with 2 drops of nettle tincture morning and evening.

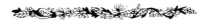

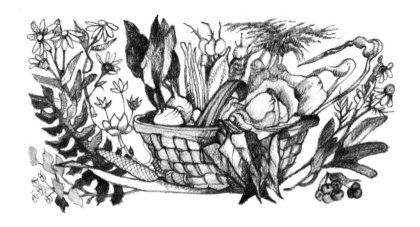

8

SKIN DISORDERS AND INJURIES

"With every occurrence of a rash, sore, eczema, or psoriasis, our body is crying for help," Pilar says. "These skin ailments are sure signs that organs responsible for excretion cannot cope with toxins in the system."

According to the Gypsy healer, suppressing skin disorders with medication or salves is useless.

"This is the only way the body can cleanse itself, since it has no alternative. Take away the body's ability to cleanse itself, and toxicity will increase, sometimes resulting in serious organic damage."

Since skin disorders are often aggravated by improper nutrition, Pilar has developed a diet that she uses with great success (see p. 80, Pilar's Healthy Skin Diet).

71

Abscesses and Flesh Wounds

PILAR'S POULTICE

black elderberry leaves
wild garlic
fresh aloe vera

Cover a piece of gauze with a salve made from ½ handful of black elderberry leaves, 7 wild garlic leaves, and a few drops of aloe vera "juice." Apply to the abscess and leave it for not more than 2 hours. If necessary, repeat the application after three hours.

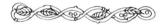

CABBAGE BANDAGE

Use 1 leaf of fresh, organically grown savoy cabbage. Rinse the leaf well, and rub it gently between your hands to make it soft and pliable. Carefully place the cabbage leaf over the abscess. If necessary, cover it with an ordinary bandage. Allow the leaf to remain in place until all toxins have been drawn out. That may take as long as 12 to 24 hours. Replace the leaf if it turns brownish-black in color or looks unsightly. Substitute red cabbage when savoy cabbage is unavailable.

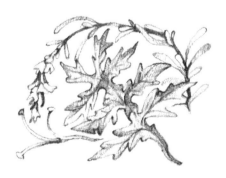

Acne

YARROW TEA

wild teasel roots
common yarrow blossoms

Harvest wild teasel roots after the first full moon in the fall. Clean, cut, and air dry teasel in a shady location. Cover a handful of roots with a quart of cold water, and bring to a boil for 10 minutes. Remove them from heat. Put 1 handful of yarrow blossoms in a separate pot, and pour the hot liquid over them. Allow the tea to steep in a covered pot for 15 minutes; strain the mixture through a gauze cloth.

Every day, morning and evening, sip one cup of tea. In addition, be sure that you are regular. Eat lots of fresh vegetables—particularly good are nettle leaves eaten like spinach.

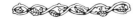

LAVENDER–ARNICA VINEGAR

lavender blossoms
arnica blossoms
apple vinegar

Mix 2 handfuls of lavender blossoms, 1 handful of arnica blossoms, and 1 quart of apple vinegar. Allow the mixture to steep in the sun for 13 days. Shake the container well morning and evening. On the 14th day, strain through a gauze cloth; fill a bottle that can be tightly sealed.

Add the Lavender–Arnica Vinegar to your wash water, or apply it with a cotton swab to the affected area of the skin.

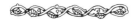

NETTLE TEA

Cover 1 handful of nettle leaves with boiling water, and steep for 10 minutes.

Drink 1 cup of nettle tea two to three times a day.

73

Bruises

With black-and-blue marks and other bruises, swelling can be kept down if the affected area is covered with a potato slice immediately after injury. You may also use Whole Arnica Tincture. For a black eye, apply potato slices to closed eyelids. Layering sliced potatoes on the skin helps soothe sunburn.

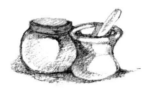

Swelling

BLOSSOM OIL

extra virgin olive oil
chamomile blossoms
arnica blossoms
comfrey

In an earthenware pot, mix 1 cup of cold-pressed (extra virgin) olive oil and 1 cup each of comfrey, chamomile blossoms, and arnica blossoms. Stir for 10 minutes. Add 1 more cup of olive oil. Cover the pot with a lid, and allow the mixture to steep for 28 days, a moon cycle, stirring once daily for 5 minutes. Filter the oil through a gauze cloth, and pour it into a brown glass container. Cover tightly and do not expose to light.

Use blossom oil compresses on bruises, subcutaneous hemorrhages, skin rashes, and stretch marks from pregnancy. This oil is also very effective for treating rheumatism, gout, and arthritis.

ARNICA BLOSSOM TINCTURE

arnica blossoms

dry white wine

180 proof alcohol

Add 1 handful of arnica blossoms to 1 cup of dry white wine, and add 1 cup of alcohol. Seal the container tightly. Allow the blossom mixture to rest for a month. Strain the mixture through a gauze cloth, and pour the tincture into bottles that can be tightly sealed.

Use the tincture for liniments and compresses on sprains or sore joints. This tincture may also be used for disinfecting wounds.

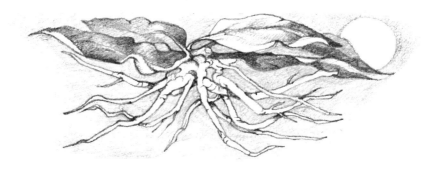

Eczema

ROOT JUICE

Grind 1 handful each of conch grass roots, nettle roots, and dandelion roots with mortar and pestle. To extract the juice, press the ground roots through a gauze cloth.

Take 1 teaspoon of fresh juice three times daily. This juice is effective for skin ulcers and insect bites.

Boils

BURDOCK ROOT TEA

burdock roots
nettle leaves
garlic cloves, crushed

Grind 1 handful of burdock roots with mortar and pestle and pour 1 quart of cold water over them. Allow the roots to steep overnight, and in the morning; boil for 5 minutes. Pour the boiling-hot mixture over ½ handful of nettle leaves. Steep in a covered pot for 15 minutes. Strain through a gauze cloth, and add 2 crushed garlic cloves.

Sip 1 cup of tea before meals three times a day. This tea is also recommended for acne, eczema, and sycosis.

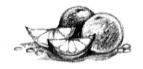

BURDOCK ROOT MUSH

burdock roots
healing earth
apple vinegar

Cut 1 handful of burdock roots into small pieces. In an earthenware pot pour water over the roots, cover the pot, and steep overnight. Bring the mixture to a boil, and simmer for 15 minutes. Cool and strain.

Mix the healing earth and the liquid to form a paste; then apply it to affected area. After half an hour, remove the dried earth with cold water and apple vinegar. This paste is also recommended for acne, eczema, and sycosis.

Foot Perspiration

ENGLISH OAK BARK CONCENTRATE

English oak bark
marigold blossoms

Cover 1 handful of English oak bark with about 2 quarts of cold water, cover, and bring to a boil. Boil until half the liquid has evaporated. Keep the pot covered and allow the oak bark to cool. Add ½ handful of marigold blossoms, stirring carefully with a wooden spoon. Steep, covered, for 13 hours. Strain through a gauze cloth.

Use the concentrate morning and evening for washing feet. Let the skin air dry; do not use a towel.

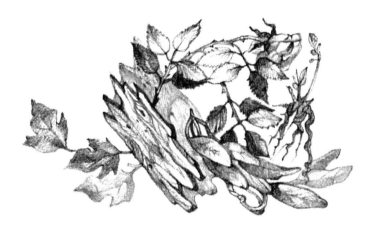

Skin Rashes and Blemishes

OYSTER SHELL POWDER

Crush oyster shells with mortar and pestle until pulverized. Take a pinch (tip of a teaspoon) of powder three times a day.

Insect Bites

THYME VINEGAR

thyme
apple vinegar
wild garlic leaves or cloves

Mix 1 handful of thyme and 1 pint of apple vinegar in a clear bottle that can be tightly sealed. Steep for one moon in a warm place or in the sun, if possible. Shake well every morning and evening. After half a moon (2 weeks), cut up 7 wild garlic leaves, and add to the mixture. If wild garlic is unavailable, crush 7 ordinary garlic cloves, and add to the mixture. After another half moon (2 weeks), strain and pour the vinegar into dark bottles. Seal tightly.

Apply Thyme Vinegar to the affected area several times a day. The vinegar will relieve itching and is also recommended for infected insect bites.

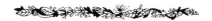

Corns

HOUSELEEK JUICE

Crush genuine houseleek leaves (*Sempervivum tectorum*) and extract the juice.

Apply fresh juice to the corn; then cover the area with a slightly crushed whole leaf, securing it gently with a bandage as necessary.

Shingles and Fever Blisters

PEPPERMINT–ROSEMARY TINCTURE

Combine 1 tablespoon of peppermint oil, 1 teaspoon of rosemary oil, and 5 tablespoons of 90 proof alcohol. Shake well.

Apply the tincture to the affected area three to five times daily.

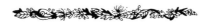

Skin Nourishment

NETTLE JUICE–YEAST

Divide 1¾ ounces of baker's or dried yeast into seven portions. Just before taking a portion of the yeast, add 1 teaspoon of fresh (if possible) nettle juice.

Take seven times daily for one moon cycle (28 days).

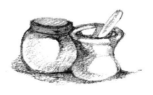

WATERMELON JUICE

After the Nettle Juice–Yeast regimen, drink one glass of freshly squeezed watermelon juice three times a day before meals for one moon cycle (28 days).

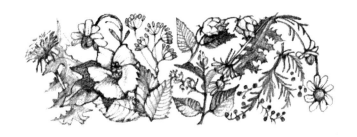

For Problem Skin

PILAR'S HEALTHY SKIN DIET

Breakfast: Drink one glass of freshly squeezed watermelon, carrot, or celery juice. Eat ½ handful of wheat germ, mixed with the juice of half a lemon, and one to two spoonfuls of honey.

If possible, add a fresh fig to the wheat germ or eat it separately. Chew two almonds, mixing them well with a sufficient amount of saliva.

Lunch: Eat only raw salad. Choose from watercress, dandelion, chickweed, sorrel, wild or regular garlic, wild rampion, garden radish, red-leaf lettuce, endive, romaine lettuce, chicory, tomatoes, carrots, cucumbers, Italian parsley, and other fresh herbs, *except* sage.

If fresh wild garlic is unavailable, use regular garlic. Garlic must be eaten every day. All other salad ingredients are exchangeable and may be used to your liking. Cut up wild garlic—even the blossoms may be eaten—or substitute 2 garlic cloves. Crush the garlic to a smooth consistency with sea salt, and add to a salad dressing of olive oil and lemon juice. Use only olive oil—no other oil—for the dressing. Add lemon juice a drop at a time to the oil and use only sea salt (not table salt) for seasoning. Do not use table salt under any circumstances.

Drink a glass of water or a glass of red wine with your meal. If you choose wine, eat one or two slices of coarse whole wheat bread with your salad.

For dessert eat a fig.

Afternoon Snack: slowly chew 3 almonds, using lots of saliva.

Dinner: Eat only vegetables that have been steamed *al dente.* Choose any of these vegetables: spinach, tomatoes, beans, carrots, red beets, cauliflower, brussels sprouts, savoy cabbage, zucchini, eggplant, artichokes, onions, mangel roots (silver beet), garlic, turnips. Season only with olive oil, sea salt, and herbs. If desired, you may also serve two boiled potatoes.

These herbs are suggested for seasoning: basil, chervil, dill, fennel, savory, thyme, parsley, chives, rosemary, lemon balm, marjoram, lovage, borage, garden cress, and tarragon.

Drink a cup of dry white wine or red wine.

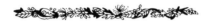

Psoriasis

HEALING PLANT SALAD

Blanch young pale green nettle leaves to avoid stinging. Mix with watercress, dandelion, and chevril. If these ingredients are not available, other herbs may be substituted. Eat as a salad or blend for a tea.

Eat the salad or drink a cup of tea daily. Sunshine also helps reduce psoriasis.

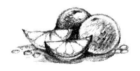

BARK COMPRESS

Mix ½ handful each of willow bark, English oak bark, and linseed. Pulverize with mortar and pestle; then add hot water to make a paste. Add fruit vinegar and Arnica Blossom Tincture (see recipe p. 75).

Apply the paste to a woolen cloth and cover affected areas.

Sunburn

ALOE VERA OIL

Add 1 pint of olive oil, a drop at a time, to 2 liqueur glasses of freshly squeezed aloe vera juice, using a wooden spoon.

The oil may be rubbed over your entire body. This oil also helps prevent insect bites and relieves the pain of burn wounds. For burns, apply the oil directly to the burn site.

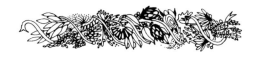

Wounds

HEDGE NETTLE WINE

hedge nettle roots and leaves
red wine
chamomile blossoms

Cut 1 handful of hedge nettle roots into small pieces, mix with 1 handful of hedge nettle leaves, and add 1 litre of red wine. Simmer in an earthenware or enamel pot for 15 minutes; then steep for 5 minutes more. Pour the liquid over ½ handful of chamomile blossoms. Allow the mixture to cool; strain through a gauze cloth.

Soak cotton or gauze in the Hedge Nettle Wine, and apply to the injury. Repeat this treatment several times. However, do not begin this treatment until every possible sign of the wound's infection has been healed.

Difficult Healing Wounds

BRIDE-OF-THE-SUN SALVE

1 handful wild garlic	9 lavender blossoms
1 cup marigold blossoms	1 cup goat butter, olive
9 rosemary blossoms	oil, or neutral base

Use olive oil or goat butter melted over a low flame for a base. But if olive oil is used, the salve will remain liquid. If you find that objectionable, use a neutral salve base (purchased at a pharmacy or health food store).

Carefully mix pot marigold blossoms, rosemary blossoms, and lavender blossoms into the base with a wooden spoon. Use only earthenware or enamel containers. Allow the mixture to simmer for 3 minutes. Remove from heat and allow to cool. Then, cover and store in a cool place. The next day, heat the salve over a very low flame once more, stirring gently for 7 minutes. Cool to body temperature and strain through a gauze cloth. Fill a glass or earthenware container, and store, tightly covered, in a cool, dark place.

Apply a thin film (repeat treatment rather than using a heavy application) of the salve to the wound.

This salve is recommended for boils, scar tissue, infections, insect bites, and diaper rash.

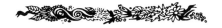

Burns

BEAR'S BREECH COMPRESS

Apply gently crushed bear's breech leaves to the affected area. A bear's breech paste may also be used. Apply the paste to a linen cloth and cover the affected area.

Although bear's breech grows primarily around the Mediterranean, some plants may survive the winter in other climates.

Sprains

COMFREY–ROSEMARY BALSAM

2 handfuls comfrey roots	3 cups olive oil
1 handful rosemary	1 handful beeswax

Gather comfrey roots during the first new moon night following the summer solstice. Clean the roots and cut them into small pieces. Add olive oil to the comfrey roots and rosemary, and place mixture in a double boiler with cold water. Stir constantly and vigorously, but do not allow mixture to come to a boil. Simmer for 13 minutes. Then, cool to body temperature, and strain through gauze, squeezing the cloth as necessary to retain the viscous substance of the comfrey in the final salve. Melt beeswax in a double boiler. While stirring the wax, add the oil, one drop at a time. Cool. If the mixture is too runny, add more liquefied beeswax.

Apply the balsam-like substance to the affected area.

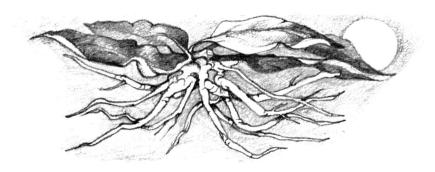

Puffy Skin

POTATO MASK

Scrub well and clean 2 to 3 potatoes. Grate for the potato mask. Apply the grated potato paste to the skin. Relax for 13 minutes. Then remove the mask and cleanse with Pilar's Rosewater–Almond Milk Lotion (see p. 86).

Cellulite

ARNICA–MARIGOLD OIL

1 handful arnica blossoms
1 handful marigold
blossoms

1 lemon rind, grated
extra virgin olive oil

Remove the petals from 1 handful each of fresh arnica blossoms and marigold blossoms, making sure that no parasites are hiding on the petals. Place the yellow petals in a clear container. Add the grated lemon rind. Carefully mix ingredients with a wooden spoon or your fingers—avoid contact with metal. Fill the glass container halfway with dry ingredients, and fill the remainder with olive oil.

Place the container in the sun for one moon cycle (28 days), shaking it every third day. Then, strain the contents and fill a dark glass container.

Use as a skin care lotion after a bath or as a massage oil. Arnica–Marigold Oil is also a good sun protection oil.

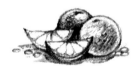

Wrinkles

PILAR'S REJUVENATING CREAM

bear's breech leaves
almond oil

Chop on a board like parsley 1 handful of bear's breech leaves. Place chopped leaves into an earthenware or porcelain container. Add 1 tablespoon of almond oil and mix well.

Apply this cream to affected area—face, neck, hands, arms, legs—for an hour. Then remove with Pilar's Rosewater–Almond Milk Lotion (see below).

Make-Up Remover and Skin Cleanser

PILAR'S ROSEWATER–ALMOND MILK LOTION

almonds
French rose blossoms
orange blossoms
Whole Arnica Tincture

Grind 1 handful of almonds with mortar and pestle. Mix 2 handfuls of French rose blossoms, and 1 teaspoon of orange blossoms. Place the blossoms in an earthenware pot, and add 1 pint of boiling water. Cover the pot and let steep for one hour. Allow liquid to cool. Add a few drops of this liquid to ground almonds in the mortar, and work the paste into a fine consistency.

Then place almond paste in an earthenware or porcelain bowl. Stirring constantly, add first a few drops of blossom liquid to almond paste, and increase the amount gradually. Pour into a clear glass container, and add 3 drops of Whole Arnica Tincture (see p. 95). Allow contents to rest in the sun for one day. Strain through a gauze cloth and fill dark bottles.

Use this lotion to remove make-up and cleanse skin. Use a cotton puff to apply the lotion to your face and neck for 3 minutes. Then remove the lotion with a clean cotton puff and clear water. This lotion works well for all skin types.

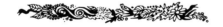

Forehead and Neck Wrinkles

PILAR'S QUINCE COMPRESS

Rub 1 handful of quince fruit with a cloth to remove the fuzz covering the skin. Cut quince into thin slices and air dry in the shade. Place the dried fruit with 2 twigs of rosemary with blossoms and 1 lavender twig with blossoms in a clear bottle. Fill the bottle with alcohol and seal tightly. Place the bottle for 13 days in the sun; shake 3 times each day. Strain through a gauze cloth and store in dark bottles.

Apply in a compress to the forehead and neck for 13 minutes. Relax—listen to music and think about wonderful experiences from the past or those you hope will come.

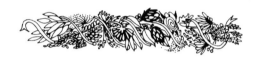

Warts

WILD GARLIC JUICE

At midnight during a full moon, apply fresh wild garlic juice to the wart. If wild garlic is unavailable, substitute freshly squeezed juice from domestic garlic cloves. Make sure the warts, after applying the juice several times, are exposed to direct moonlight in open air for 3 minutes.

During these 3 minutes, concentrate on the thought that your body has stopped nurturing the warts; so, they have to die. This charm, used with both children and adults, is helpful:

> *Nasty wart, go away!*
> *Part from me.*
> *And do not stay.*
> *Nasty wart, go away!*

Freckles

GARLIC–VINEGAR PASTE

Crush 3 garlic cloves with mortar and pestle to form a paste. Add fruit vinegar one drop at a time to create a pliable paste.

Apply the paste morning and evening to affected areas for 13 minutes. Remove and apply Bride-of-the-Sun Salve (p. 83). This paste is also effective against age spots.

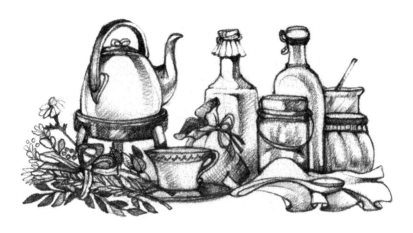

—9—
RHEUMATISM AND CHRONIC PAIN

Gypsies have few problems with chronic, painful muscle and joint diseases known as rheumatism.

Modern medicine has divided these many varied diseases according to their individual symptoms and given each a separate name—such as, arthritis, polyarthritis, spondylitis, and osteochondritis. Usually, allopathic medicine is helpless in treating these diseases in spite of its meticulous categorizations of these ailments. In the Western world, rheumatic illnesses have become widespread. Unfortunately, the number of people afflicted with these chronic diseases seems to be steadily increasing.

Are rheumatic diseases unavoidable in our civilization, and must people afflicted with them live with them for better or worse?

Pilar believes, "Rheumatism can be cured if one chooses the right approach to the illness."

"Generally, we are most vulnerable to these illnesses from October through February." As a preventive and certainly for all those already suffering from a rheumatic disease, Pilar recommends Lentil Juice Cure (see p. 91). "Anyone willing to follow this treatment for at least 6 months will marvel at the result. Nature often surprises us with the effectiveness of simple remedies."

For rheumatism Pilar advises that people first discontinue any exposure to synthetically produced medication. "To suppress the symptoms makes no sense and will only place patients in a vicious cycle. Patients must come to terms with their illness and accept it. This is true for every illness, as I have said. A disease is the body's cry for help to the afflicted demanding *change!*"

Pilar considers rheumatism to be caused by waste products and toxins that have accumulated in the system. The body suffers from too much acid. This situation may have developed over several years until adverse conditions like sun spots and changes in weather trigger symptoms, and the illness becomes serious.

Pilar suggests that people with rheumatism "mentally wish away and thereby help your body rid itself of toxins that have accumulated! Ready yourself for the process, and be patient. You cannot repair your body like a car; you have to fight the cause of the illness, not the obvious symptoms.

"Confine yourself to bed rest for two or three weeks. I know it is boring and bothersome. But what are a few weeks in exchange for better health?"

Pilar also offers this general advice: Use only natural, untreated cotton sheets. Use comforters and blankets made from natural fibres like cotton, wool, or sheepskin. Avoid any synthetic fibres for underwear or clothes.

Fast for at least 13 days, and drink juice from raw potatoes mixed with 1 tablespoon of healing earth. Also drink 1 tablespoon of nettle juice three times a day. Carrot juice is also allowed.

Help rid your body of waste products and toxins with a sweating cure by drinking a perspiration-inducing tea, Pilar's Rheumatism Tea I (see p. 93), every three hours or just twice a day, depending on how much tea you can tolerate.

Listen to music and try to sleep. If it is hard to induce perspiration, add more blankets, even in summer. Place a hot-water bottle on your feet.

After sweating, wash with lukewarm water to which a twig of rosemary herb has been added. Dry the body quickly. Use Blossom Oil (see p. 74) for all painful areas. If necessary, use Blossom Oil in compresses.

Do not forget the Lentil Juice Cure.

To escape the cycle of illness, follow a strict diet. "You will be rewarded with a feeling of freshness, youthfulness, and vigor. I know it's hard to let habits go, but you may be able to gently return to some of your former ways, after you have overcome your illness. But don't overdo it. Watch for signals the body sends. I think the price for regaining one's joy for life is not too high."

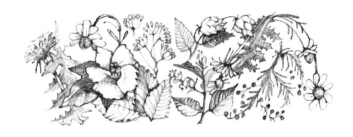

Gout

LENTIL JUICE CURE

Soak 1 teaspoon of lentils in a covered pot overnight in ½ cup of water. Strain in the morning.

Drink the lentil juice in the morning on an empty stomach. Throw away the lentils. Continue this treatment for at least 6 months.

Lumbago and Sciatica

BARK TEA

willow bark
birch bark
blind nettle

Mix 1 handful each of willow bark, birch bark, and blind nettle. Pour boiling water over the dry ingredients, and steep for 3 hours. Strain through a gauze cloth.

Sip 1 cup of the tea at body temperature three times a day. Bark tea may be sweetened with honey.

For a compress, soak and wring out a cotton cloth in the tea, and apply to the painful area. Cover the compress with another cotton cloth, and wrap the area in a woolen cloth to prevent cold air from reaching the area. Also cover yourself with a blanket.

SAINT-JOHN'S-WORT OIL

Place Saint-John's-wort blossoms in a clear glass container, and pour 1 quart of olive oil over them. Seal tightly and allow the blossom mixture to steep for a moon cycle (28 days) in full sun. Strain and fill a dark bottle or glass container with the oil.

The oil may be used as a liniment. For wound treatment, apply a small piece of cotton soaked in the oil. This oil is also recommended for neuralgia, tennis elbow, neck pain, muscle spasm, painful wounds, sunburn, and painful scar tissue.

Caution: Exposure to sun just after handling Saint-John's-Wort Oil may cause skin blotches.

Rheumatism

PILAR'S RHEUMATISM TEA I

½ handful European ash bark

½ handful European ash seeds

½ handful European ash leaves

1 licorice root, half-thumb width

¼ handful peppermint leaves

1 tablespoon cornflower blossoms

1 tablespoon marigold blossoms

Grind European ash bark with mortar and pestle. Cut European ash seeds and leaves, licorice root, peppermint leaves, cornflower blossoms, and marigold blossoms into small pieces. Mix and store in a container that seals tightly.

Place 1 handful of the mixture in an earthenware pot, and add 1 quart of boiling water. Steep, covered, for 15 minutes. Strain through gauze cloth.

Sip 1 cup of tea, as hot as possible, every three hours. This tea will induce sweating, lower fever, and decrease infections. Stay in bed, and have a cotton terrycloth towel and fresh sheets ready. Avoid drafts.

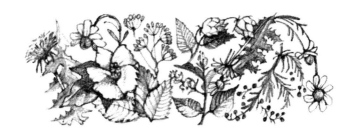

PILAR'S RHEUMATISM TEA II

European ash leaves
black elderberry bark
pine needles

Cut 1 handful of black elderberry bark into small pieces. Place the bark with 1 handful of European ash leaves and ½ handful of pine needles in an earthenware pot, and add 1 quart of boiling water. Boil for 3 minutes. Cover and steep for 15 minutes. Strain through gauze cloth.

Sip not more than 2 cups a day of the tea. Use this tea if ingredients for Pilar's Rheumatism Tea I are unavailable. A variation on this recipe, below, makes a soothing bath.

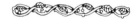

BATH EXTRACT FOR RHEUMATISM

Add 1 pint of cold water to 2 handfuls of European ash leaves, 1 handful of black elderberry bark, and ½ handful of pine leaves. Bring to just below boiling point in an open earthenware pot. Simmer for 20 minutes. Strain and add the extract to warm bath water.

Stay in the tub for 20 minutes. Shower briefly with cold water, dry the skin well, and rest at least 20 minutes.

Pilar's Diet for Rheumatism

You may eat lots of potatoes, steamed with the skin, or the raw juice; raw root vegetables or their juice—carrots, beets, celery, viper's-grass roots; olive oil; butter; cottage cheese; yogurt; wheat germ; dandelion leaves; watercress; fresh wild garlic (substitute regular garlic if unavailable); 6 well-chewed almonds daily; goat cheese; and 3 teaspoons daily of nettle juice freshly squeezed. Continue this diet while taking the Lentil Juice Cure.

Also drink Heal-Everything Tonic (p. 20), and Gitano Bitter (p. 22) to increase stamina.

Do *not* eat white bread, cakes, jams, fruits, canned food, honey, onions, sugar, table salt, processed food, meats, cold cuts, bacon, or ham. Also do not drink coffee, black tea, or alcohol. Quit smoking.

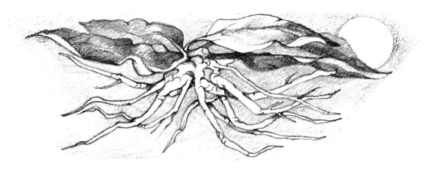

Rheumatic Pain

WHOLE ARNICA TINCTURE

arnica blossoms, leaves, and roots
140 proof alcohol

Harvest the arnica plant—blossoms, leaves, and roots—during the night of the new moon that immediately follows the summer solstice.

Wash the whole plant. Remove its petals from the base of the blossoms, because that's where insects like to hide, and carefully clean the base. Cut the plant, including the roots, into small pieces. Cover with alcohol, and allow it to rest in direct sun for a moon cycle. Shake the container well once a day. Strain the tincture on the 29th day and pour it into a dark bottle for storage.

Add 1 tablespoon of the tincture to 2 cups of water. Soak a gauze cloth in the mixture, and apply it to the painful area.

Diluted Whole Arnica Tincture may be applied externally. It is recommended for headaches, edemas, and bruises as well as disinfecting cuts and wounds—use in a compress.

95

"I want to plead that readers not prepare this remedy themselves, because the last arnica remaining in the mountains would surely be destroyed. I know arnica is legally protected in many places. But I also know only too well that laws are not very effective when understanding, insight, and the will to accept them are missing." So it's best to buy whole arnica tincture in stores. Instructions for the tincture are included here because they are typical of the way Gypsies prepare their remedies.

The plant's list of benefits is almost as long as the list of common names for *arnica*—arnica root, common arnica, leopardsbane, mountain arnica, mountain tobacco, wolfsbane.

Europeans once considered arnica a holy, mystical plant. They believed arnica, like mistletoe, would bring blessings, and they used it during summer solstice rituals. Gypsies have long known its healing powers. They consider arnica to have the power of wolves—wild, courageous, and unpredictable animals that are always kind toward their own.

"If you want to gain the benefits and blessings of the arnica plant, you must approach it with reverence and respect. If you pick it with thoughtlessness or lack of feelings, or overdose on its good energies, arnica will 'bare her teeth' with uncomfortable side effects. People who understand the characteristics of arnica also know how to avoid those dangers," Pilar says. She calls arnica *Lobocito del Sol,* "Little Sun-Wolf."

The orthodox medical community once labeled arnica an aphrodisiac. Pilar says "it is quite possible that 'Little Sun-Wolf' might have just such an effect since it stimulates the whole person and provides courage."

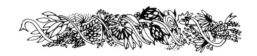

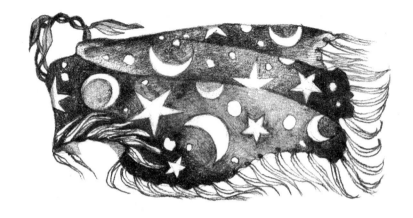

—10—

INSOMNIA AND NERVOUS STRESS

Black clouds loom as a storm brews and uncomfortably hot air in the trailer camp hangs heavily with dust. The birds are silent. Women busily gather clothes from the clothesline—expansive skirts artfully patched from remnants, puffy sleeved blouses, patchwork pillow cases, blue jeans, checkered shirts. Men roll up canvases protecting the trailers from the sun. Children run about excitedly. Little Rodrigo stands at the edge of the camp peeing, creating a rainbow-colored arch. I ask Pilar to talk about fear.

"You are asking about fear." She leans back on the chair in her trailer. "A difficult subject."

"Why, Pilar?" I ask. "We've already talked about so many things that seemed much more difficult."

"Yes and no. Fear is so omnipresent, untouchable, boundless. It seems to follow us with silent steps, like a bad spirit. Those who insist they are never afraid are lying. Or they are monsters!

"Fear is part of life. But you Payos are ashamed when you experience fear, as if it were a sin. So, the result of fear is depression, insomnia, and hopelessness. You cannot escape these unless you face the fear."

The Gypsy healer considers it dangerous to suppress fear with psychiatric drugs: "That will not resolve anything, only increase a vicious cycle." As with other illnesses, Pilar advises that we treat not the symptoms but address the reason for suffering.

"Talk about what bothers you—it is liberating. And you will find people who understand you. Fear is not something we have to be ashamed of. For instance, is it not normal to be afraid of the destruction that threatens our Mother Earth?

"Fears should be discussed openly—with anyone you trust. This might give a friend the courage to talk about his own fear. Both of you will be stronger as a result.

"As with everything else in life, fear also has to be approached positively. Fear is not our enemy. Fear can be our friend. Fear makes animals attentive and careful. Depending on their predisposition, they will either save themselves by running, or they will fight."

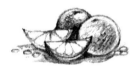

But humans must face the fear. "The first step to healing is to say 'yes' to yourself, accept the good and the bad parts of yourself." Nightmares, depression, insomnia, and nervous illnesses are a sign that you need to reorganize your life.

"Every thought has psychological and physical effects. Force yourself to think positively. Find what's positive in everything that happens to you. That way, you turn fear around and make it work for you!"

Write down everything on a piece of paper—negative emotions and thoughts you want to change. "Then, burn the paper, lie down, close your eyes, and listen to music."

Headaches

BANISH PAIN TONIC

willow bark

Saint-John's-wort

Pulverize willow bark with mortar and pestle, and cut Saint-John's-wort into small pieces. For each cup of tonic, mix 2 teaspoons of willow bark powder and ¼ teaspoon of Saint-John's-wort. It's okay to prepare 3 to 4 cups, a day's ration, in advance and gently warm the liquid when needed.

Place the mixture in an earthenware or enamel pot, cover with water, and simmer for 13 minutes. After it cools, strain the liquid through gauze.

Sip 3 to 4 cups of this tonic daily. It may be sweetened with honey. This tonic is recommended for migraine headaches, painful joints, flu, and fever and for relieving soreness.

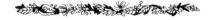

Nervousness

VALERIAN WINE

2 handfuls valerian roots

1 clove

1 orange rind, organically grown

1 rosemary twig

1 litre dry white wine

Cut valerian root into small pieces, and place them in a large clear glass container. Add the clove, the grated orange rind, and rosemary twig. Pour the dry white wine over the dry mixture. Seal the container tightly and allow to steep for one moon cycle (28 days). Then strain through gauze cloth, store in a bottle, and seal tightly.

Drink 1 liqueur glass three times a day.

Pilar's Valerian Wine is recommended for nervous heart condition, faintness, nervous headache, menopausal symptoms, stomach pain, intestinal cramps, colics, gallbladder disorders, strengthening the nervous system, and stimulating circulation.

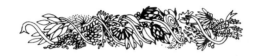

Insomnia

NINE-HERB FRAGRANT SLEEPING PILLOW

1 handful Saint-John's-wort leaves and blossoms
1 handful valerian blossoms
1 handful balm leaves
1 handful Roman chamomile leaves
2 handfuls bird's-foot trefoil
½ handful orange blossoms
1 handful rose blossoms
1 handful lavender blossoms
3 orange rinds, finely grated

Mix Saint-John's-wort leaves and blossoms, valerian blossoms, lemon balm leaves, chamomile leaves, rose blossoms, and lavender blossoms. Add bird's-foot trefoil, orange blossoms, and finely grated orange rind. Mix ingredients well, and put them inside a cotton pillow case.

Place the pillow under or atop your regular pillow. Your body temperature releases the fragrances of the leaves and blossoms. Replace the herb contents of your pillow every 2 to 3 months. This pillow calms nerves, helps you fall asleep, and induces deep, restful sleep.

PILLOW FOR TEETHING CHILDREN AND SICK ADULTS

1 handful valerian roots, chopped
1 handful German chamomile
1 handful sage
1 handful rosemary
1 handful male fern, chopped
1 handful lemon balm
13 arnica flowers
13 mistletoe berries

Mix German chamomile, sage, rosemary, lemon balm, chopped male fern, and chopped valerian roots. Add arnica flowers and mistletoe berries. Place ingredients inside a cotton pillow case.

Place this fragrant pillow under your pillow. The herb pillow is nice for teething children, since it relieves pain and helps the child relax and fall asleep. Change pillow contents every 2 months.

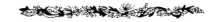

SEVEN HERB TEA

2 tablespoons Saint-John's-wort leaves
2 tablespoons lemon balm leaves
1 tablespoon valerian roots, chopped
1 teaspoon orange blossoms
1 teaspoon passionflower blossoms
1 tablespoon bird's-foot trefoil blossoms *or* sweet clover (melitot) blossoms

Mix Saint-John's-wort, lemon balm leaves, chopped valerian roots, orange blossoms, passionflower blossoms, and either bird's-foot trefoil blossoms or sweet clover blossoms. Use 1 tablespoon of the dry mixture for each cup of tea. Cover with boiling water and allow the tea to steep for 13 minutes.

Drink 1 cup of tea before retiring.

Psychosomatic Illnesses

SOUL-REFRESHING TONIC

Saint-John's-wort leaves and blossoms
90 proof alcohol

Gather the fresh shoots of Saint-John's-wort between the summer solstice and St. John's Day (June 21 and 24) at sunrise. Remove the blossoms and leaves, and place them in a dark glass container that can be sealed tightly. Cover with 90 proof alcohol. Steep for one moon cycle (28 days) in a dark place. Shake every third day. After one moon, strain the contents through a gauze cloth and fill dark dropper bottles. Close lids tightly.

Give ½ liqueur glass of Soul-Refresher Tonic to a person in shock due to an accident. Otherwise, take 20 drops daily.

Pilar says: "Saint-John's-wort herb flows through the whole body, making it receptive to cosmic energies. After taking the tonic, do not expose yourself to intense sunlight. White skin blotches may develop."

Pilar recommends Soul-Refreshing Tonic for fear, emotional pain, melancholy, depression, shock after an accident, headaches after concussion, and for calming nerves and heart palpitation.

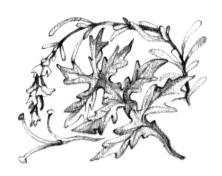

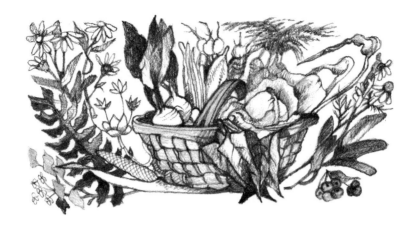

11

LOVE POTIONS AND SENSUALITY

About love, "an old man cannot be transformed in an instant into a fiery lover simply by gulping down a cup of my aphrodisiac. It might be possible, but many ingredients are necessary to make this happen—mood, devotion to one's partner, emotional state, ability to trust, soft light, music—the whole range of positive influences that lend fantasies wings.

"The power of love is closest to the fountain of life. Of all things, love is what keeps us young, flexible, joyful, and healthy. Love brings us close to life itself. But love and sex must be approached with deep respect, reverence, and an attitude of joyful play. This vital spark does not depend on age. Rather, it is a matter of a radiant, positive attitude toward life."

Gypsies do not lose their close connection to Mother Earth's positive energies. Two plants native to Asia Minor with strong eroticizing effects were brought to Europe: lovage—also called sea parsley, pleasure stick, love stem, or nine-stem—and jim-sonweed.

Use the fresh blossoms, leaves, stems, and roots of lovage to add spark and spice to cooked food and salads. But lovage, including the roots, can also be ground up with mortar and pestle.

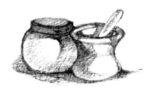

About the aphrodisiac jimsonweed, Pilar says: "Look at the pollen of this plant in bloom—you will agree that it has an uncanny resemblance to a proud phallus. Ground jimsonweed seeds make you cheerful and receptive to lovemaking. But, de-termining a proper dosage is difficult and must be precisely measured for each individual. I cannot give approximate in-struction without committing a sin."

During witch hunts in the 17th century jimsonweed was called the thorn apple or devil's apple. A 17th century docu-ment warns: "With this weed one can make a wench do any-thing that one pleases; there is no other herb on earth so dan-gerous which can bring about—although in a natural way—so much evil."

Pilar warns: "The seeds are dangerous and should never be taken internally. I prepare a salve to be used only externally. It has a stimulating effect since it is absorbed through the skin."

Aphrodisiac

LOVAGE TEA

Grind 1 handful lovage blossoms, leaves, stems, and roots into a powder with mortar and pestle. For a cup of tea, pour boiling water over 1 tablespoon of powder, and let steep for 13 minutes.

Both the man and the woman should sip this tea slowly.

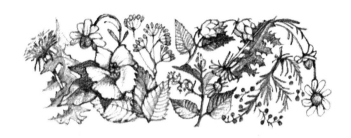

PILAR'S LOVE POTION

2 tablespoons muirapiranga (potent wood)
1 teaspoon damiana root (*Turnera diffusa*)
½ teaspoon yohimbe bark (*Corynanthe yohimbe*)
1 handful wheat germ
½ handful lovage
1 litre red wine

Cut muirapiranga (potent wood) and damiana root into small pieces, and add ½ teaspoon yohimbine (from yohimbe bark—*Corynanthe yohimbe*). Add wheat germ and lovage. Mix ingredients well. Pour red wine over dry ingredients. First place the container for half a moon in the sun; then for half a moon place it in a dark place. Strain through a gauze cloth.

Lovers may drink half a wine glass of the potion.

LOVE CREAM

jimsonweed seeds
pork fat or neutral base

Grind 1 teaspoon jimsonweed seeds into powder with a mortar and pestle. Mix the powder with 1 handful pork fat or neutral base (available in pharmacies or health food stores).

The man and woman apply a small amount of this cream to erotic zones, as well as the armpits, behind the knees, and around the navel.

Caution: Use the cream externally only. Jimsonweed taken internally is poisonous.

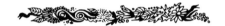

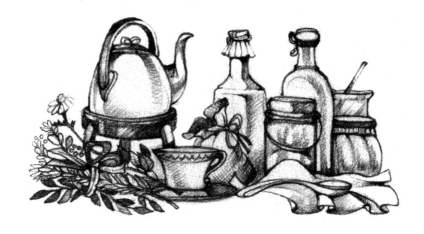

—12—
REMEDIES FOR ANIMALS

Gypsies, being close to nature, feel close to our fellow animals. They once felt particularly close to wolves. And today, since they share the forest with them, they feel a kinship with foxes, deer, and rabbits.

Two domesticated animals have been faithful companions to Gypsies in their world travels—the horse which once pulled Gypsy wagons and the dog which alerts them of danger.

Before trucks, automobiles, and trailers replaced horses and wagons, Gypsies earned a living by trading horses. Their expertise was unequaled. They could successfully treat lame animals or make an old mare sparkle with life in a short time.

Gypsies' traditional knowledge of animal husbandry earned them money. European farmers often call Gypsies to their stables when a cow or sheep falls sick, hens stop laying eggs, or geese fail to grow fat. Gypsies have seemingly miraculous salves to heal wounds, but they have kept the ingredients secret. They applied compresses to sprained ankles and bruises and swiftly healed paw, hoof, or wing.

Gypsies disinfect stables in two stages. First, they rid them of flies by hanging a bunch of the mugwort plant from the ceiling. As soon as flies attached themselves to the plant, they stuffed the plant into a bag, closed it tightly, and burned the sack outside. In the second phase, they took the animals out of the stable and closed windows and doors. They then loosely tied together 3 braids of dried garlic, 5 twigs of thyme, and 3 twigs of rosemary, and burned them slowly inside the stable. After at least 1 hour the stable would be disinfected.

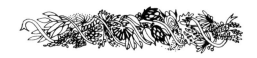

General Remedies

TO STOP BLEEDING

Mix 1 handful of rosemary and 1 tablespoon of pulverized English oak bark, and add 1 quart of boiling water. Allow to cool to body temperature. Strain the liquid and use for wound cleansing. Then apply ground rosemary to the animal's wound.

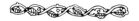

FOR INSECT AND SPIDER BITES

Crush a fresh clove of garlic in vinegar or lemon juice. Dab on the affected area. This solution should be available when needed. Prepare it in advance and store in a small bottle.

FOR EAR PARASITES

Mix linseed oil with an equal amount of olive oil. Bring to a lukewarm temperature, and with a dropper carefully add drops in the animal's ear.

FOR INTESTINAL PARASITES

Cut wild garlic into small pieces, and mix it into the animal's feed. If wild garlic is not available, use regular garlic. This preventive remedy strengthens the intestines and helps prevent colics. Dogs and cats should be given this remedy once a week.

To heal injuries, infections, bone problems, and fractures, apply Comfrey–Rosemary Balsam (see page 84), after thoroughly cleansing the affected area.

FOR ECZEMA

Grind acorns into powder and dust the affected area of the animal's skin. Also, put the animal on a three-day fast. Give it only water to drink that has been sweetened with honey to relieve the system of toxins. Continue feeding after the third day; add crushed garlic to the feed. Dosage depends on the size of the animal. For a cat, 2 cloves of garlic, perhaps mixed with milk, are sufficient.

Do not skip this part of the treatment, since it stimulates the animal's energies. If the animal refuses to eat the garlic, wrap it in a piece of its favorite food, such as meat or fish. Always use fresh garlic—never garlic powder.

FOR SCABIES AND LICE

Mix oil from the laurel tree fruit with equal parts of olive oil, and add 3 drops of rosemary oil. Rub into the animal's coat. The oil will remove parasites. In severe cases, bathe the animal before applying the oil. Do not use detergent or soap powder; use only pure soap and a rosemary herb wash instead of plain water.

FOR SPRAINS, ARTHRITIS, AND BRUISES

Dilute Whole Arnica Tincture (see page 95). Use 2 tablespoons for every pint of water. Moisten a piece of gauze, and apply it to the affected area. Secure with a bandage. Repeat every 30 minutes.

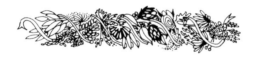

Remedies for Dogs

TO CALM A DOG IN HEAT

Take ½ handful of passionflower blossoms and add 1 quart of water. Steep for 13 minutes, strain, and add to the dog's drinking water.

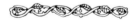

FOR DIARRHEA

Use only the flesh of the carob fruit, not the seeds, and add 1 to 2 tablespoons to food.

FOR A HEALTHY COAT

For a healthy coat and as a preventive against rheumatism, every 13th day add ¼ to ½ handful of dried, pulverized nettle to the dog's food. The amount to add depends on the animal's size. One teaspoon is enough for a small dog.

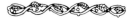

FOR RECUPERATION FROM ILLNESS

Give the dog milk to drink, with 1 pinch of nutmeg and 1 teaspoon of honey added.

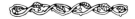

FOR CONSTIPATION

Depending on the size of the animal, give it from 1 teaspoon to 1 tablespoon of olive oil.

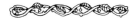

FOR BRONCHITIS

Cut a large onion into small pieces. Boil in milk until the onion is well done. Cool and sweeten with honey. Give the dog 1 to 2 cups during the day.

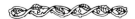

FOR OBESITY

Pulverize carob fruit with mortar and pestle, and mix into food. Feed the dog, depending on its size, 1 to 2 tablespoons of the pulverized fruit daily.

FOR WEAK HEART OR DIFFICULTY BREATHING

Cut ½ handful of valerian root into small pieces, and bring to a boil in 1 pint of water. Remove from the fire and allow the roots to steep. Strain. Add a drop of Whole Arnica Tincture (see p. 95). Give the dog 1 teaspoon every hour.

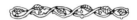

FOR PARASITES

(1) Crush 3 to 4 garlic bulbs (not cloves but whole bulbs, peeled) with mortar and pestle to make a paste. Use more for a large dog. Mix the garlic paste with milk, and add 1 teaspoon of honey. If the dog is unwilling to drink the remedy, pour the milk down the animal's throat.

(2) Mix equal amounts of olive oil and castor oil. For each tablespoon of the oil mixture, add 1 drop of pomegranate juice. Give this to the dog a half hour after the garlic milk remedy.

After this treatment, add wild garlic (regular garlic if wild garlic is unavailable) to your dog's food once a week.

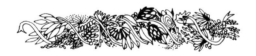

Remedies for Rabbits

Add fresh parsley to the rabbit's daily food as well as boiled, peeled, and finely chopped horse chestnuts.

FOR CONJUNCTIVITIS

Carefully wash the rabbit's eyes with a weak German chamomile tea.

FOR TYMPANITIS

Add 1 handful of garden thyme to the rabbit's food.

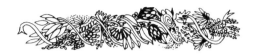

Remedies for Cats

TO CALM NERVOUS CATS

Add a pinch of passionflowers to 1 cold cup of water. Bring to a boil and remove from the fire. Allow the tonic to steep for 3 minutes; strain.

Give this to your cat instead of plain water. If necessary, add a few drops of milk.

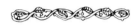

FOR A HEALTHY COAT

Once every 13 days, mix dried, finely chopped nettle leaves to the cat's food. This will also stimulate the cat's immune system.

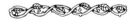

FOR COLDS AND BRONCHITIS

Pour boiling water over 1 tablespoon of eucalyptus leaves, and steep for 13 minutes. Strain and sweeten heavily with brown, unprocessed sugar. Give the cat 2 cups of tea daily.

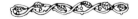

FOR CONSTIPATION

Give the cat 1 tablespoon of olive oil.

FOR DIARRHEA

Toast a loaf of white bread in the oven until it is almost burned. Scrape off the burned portions and mix into the cat's food.

Also, pour boiling water over a few artichoke leaves. Steep for 3 minutes. Strain and add 10 drops of this liquid to the food mixed with charcoal toast.

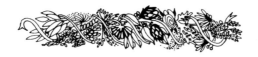

Remedies for Horses

One handful of nettle seeds, mixed daily with the feed, acts as a fountain of youth for horses. It makes them eager, they step lively, and it gives them a shimmering, silky coat and sparkling eyes.

Gypsies harvest nettle seeds in the fall. They collect seeds from both the large nettle (*Urtica dioica*) and the dwarf nettle (*Urtica urens*), species that are widespread. Seeds are air dried in the shade and stored in bags made from natural fiber.

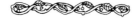

FOR CONSTIPATION

Cut up 3 pieces of carob fruits. Add 3 soft-boiled garlic bulbs. Give to the horse in two portions during the day.

FOR FEVER

Chop a bunch of parsley, and add to diluted, cold black tea. Have the horse drink this tea three times a day.

TO STIMULATE LABOR CONTRACTIONS

Just when the foal is about to be born, give the mare 13 to 21 cloves without stems. The dosage depends on the size of the horse.

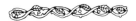

FOR COUGHS AND BRONCHITIS

Sprinkle water in the horse's feeding trough to eliminate dust. Cut 2 carrots and 2 whole garlic bulbs into small pieces. Add to the feed once a day.

Cover ½ handful each of sage and eucalyptus leaves with boiling water. Steep for 13 minutes, cool, and add 2 teaspoons of honey. Have the horse drink this cough remedy.

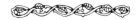

FOR DIARRHEA

Mix 1 tablespoon of pulverized English oak bark and 3 tablespoons of honey into the feed. Continue this treatment for at least three days until the horse's bowel movements are normal again.

Combine this treatment with a moderate amount of nettle seeds; about ½ handful of seeds will be enough.

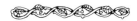

FOR RHEUMATISM

Feed the animal nettle seeds. Also feed the horse fresh young, light green nettle leaves and nettle stems. To avoid stinging, scald the leaves with boiling water.

FOR COLICS

Feed the horse equal amounts of dandelion and fennel leaves.

FOR WORMS

Place the horse on a two-day fast.

Cut 5 garlic bulbs into small pieces, add honey, and mix into the feed bran. The dosage will depend on the animal's size.

As a preventive, add to the horse's feed male fern, black elderberries, and couch grass. These herbs will be most effective when used freshly cut from the meadow.

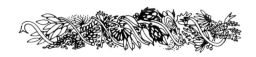

Remedies for Birds

Depending on the time of year, feed birds black elderberries, juniper, hawthorn, chickweed, fennel seeds, and flaxseeds.

Caution: Parsley and caraway seeds are poisonous for birds.

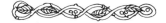

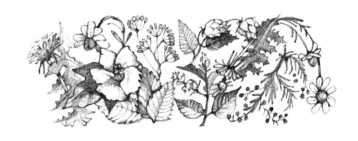

BOTANICAL NAMES
OF PLANTS

Absinthe (Wormwood)	*Artemisia absinthium*
Almond	*Prunus amygdalus*
Aloe Vera	*Aloe vera*
Angelica	*Angelica archangelica*
Anise	*Pimpinella anisum*
Arnica	*Arnica montana*
Artichoke	*Cynara scolymus*
Ash, European	*Fraxinus excelsior*
Asparagus	*Asparagus officinalis*
Bachelor's Button (Cornflower)	*Centaurea cyanus*
Basil	*Ocimum basilicum*
Bear's Breech	*Acanthus mollis*
Bear's Garlic (Wild Garlic, Wood Garlic, Ransoms)	*Allium ursinum*
Bearberry	*Arctostaphylos uva-ursi*
Beet	*Beta vulgaris*
Bergamot	*Citrus bergamia*
Birch, Silver (European White Birch)	*Betula pendula*
Bird's-Foot Trefoil	*Lotus corniculatus*
Bitter Orange	*Citrus aurantium*
Blackberry (Bramble)	*Rubus fructicosus*

Black Mulberry	*Morus nigra*
Black Mustard	*Brassica nigra*
Black Elderberry	*Sambucus nigra*
Blind Nettle (White Dead Nettle)	*Lamium album*
Borage	*Borago officinalis*
Bramble (Blackberry)	*Rubus fructicosus*
Burdock (Greater Burdock)	*Arctium lappa*
Burnet Saxifrage, Greater	*Pimpinella major*
Cabbage	*Brassica oleracea capitata*
Calamus (Sweet Flag)	*Acorus calamus*
Calendula (Pot Marigold, Common Marigold)	*Calendula officinalis*
Carob	*Ceratonia siliqua*
Carrot	*Daucus sativus carota*
Castor Bean	*Ricinus communis*
Catarrh Root (Galangal, Galanga)	*Alpina* species
Celery	*Apium graveolens*
Centaury, European	*Centaurium erythraea*
Chickweed	*Stellaria media*
Chives	*Allium schoenoprasum*
Cloves	*Syzygium aromaticum*
Cluster Pine (Maritime Pine)	*Pinus pinaster*
Coltsfoot	*Tussilago farfara*
Comfrey	*Symphytum officinale*
Common Mallow	*Malva silvestris*
Cornflower (Bachelor's Button)	*Centaurea cyanus*
Couch Grass (Quack Grass, Witch Grass)	*Agropyron repens*
Cowslip	*Primula veris*
Crocus	*Crocus* species
Cucumber	*Cucumis sativus*
Cypress	*Cypressus* species
Daisy, English	*Bellis perennis*
Dandelion	*Taraxacum officinale*
Dewcup (Lady's Mantle)	*Alchemilla vulgaris*

Dill	*Anethum graveolens*
Dog Rose	*Rosa canina*
Dwarf Nettle (Small Nettle)	*Uritca urens*
English Daisy	*Bellis perennis*
English Oak (Pedunculate Oak)	*Quercus robur*
Eucalyptus	*Eucalyptus globulus*
Eurasian Sedum (Orpine)	*Sedum telephium*
European Ash	*Fraxinus excelsior*
European Centaury	*Centaurium erythraea*
European Mistletoe (Mistletoe)	*Viscum album*
Eyebright	*Euphrasia officinalis*
Fennel	*Foeniculum vulgare*
Fenugreek	*Trigonella foenumgraecum*
Fern	*Aspidium felix-mas*
Fern, Male	*Drypopteris filix-mas*
Fig	*Ficus carica*
Fireweed (Rose Bay Willow-Herb)	*Epilobium chamaenerion angustifolium*
Flax	*Linum usitatissimum*
Florentine Iris (Orrisroot)	*Iris florentina*
French Rose	*Rosa gallica*
Fumitory	*Fumaria officinalis*
Galangal (Catarrh Root, Galanga)	*Alpina* species
Garden Cress	*Lepidium sativum*
Garden Sorrel	*Rumex acetosa*
Garlic	*Allium sativum*
Garlic, Wild (Wood Garlic, Bear's Garlic, Ransoms)	*Allium ursinum*
German (Blue) Chamomile	*Matricaria chamomilla*
Ginger (Gingerroot)	*Zingiber officinale*
Gold Heart (Ivy)	*Hedera helix*
Greater Burdock	*Arctium lappa*
Hawthorn (Common Hawthorn)	*Crataegus monogyna*
Hazel (Cobnut)	*Corylus avellana*

Hedge Nettle	*Stachys officinalis*
Hibiscus	*Hibiscus* species
Hops	*Humulus lupulus*
Horehound	*Marrubium vulgare*
Horsetail	*Equisetum* species
Houseleek	*Sempervivum tectorum*
Italian Parsley	*Petroselinum hortense*
Ivy (Gold Heart)	*Hedera helix*
Jimsonweed	*Datura stamonium*
Juniper (Common Juniper)	*Juniperus communis*
Kidney Bean	*Phaseolus vulgaris*
Lady's Mantle (Dewcup)	*Alchemilla vulgaris*
Large Nettle	*Urtica dioica*
Laurel	*Laurus nobilis*
Lavender	*Lavandula officinalis*
Lemon Balm (Melissa)	*Melissa officinalis*
Lemon	*Citrus limon*
Lentil	*Lens culinaris*
Licorice	*Glycyrrhiza glabra*
Linden	*Tilia cordata*
Long-spurred Pansy	*Viola calcarata*
Lovage	*Levisticum officinale*
Lungwort	*Pulonaria officinalis*
Male Fern	*Drypopteris filix-mas*
Marigold, Pot (Calendula, Common Marigold)	*Calendula officinalis*
Maritime Pine (Cluster Pine)	*Pinus pinaster*
Masterwort	*Peucedanum ostruthium*
Medlar	*Mespilus germanica*
Melilot (Sweet Clover)	*Melilotus officinalis*
Melissa (Lemon Balm)	*Melissa officinalis*
Mistletoe (European Mistletoe)	*Viscum album*
Mugwort	*Artemisia vulgaris*
Musk Melon	*Cucumis melo*
Mustard, Black	*Brassica nigra*
Myrtle	*Myrtus communis*
Nettle, Large	*Urtica dioica*

Nettle, Blind (White Dead Nettle)	*Lamium album*
Nettle, Dwarf (Small Nettle)	*Urtica urens*
Nipplewort	*Lapsana communis*
Nutmeg	*Myristica fragans*
Oak, English (Pendum Culate Oak)	*Quercus robur*
Oats	*Avena sativa*
Olive	*Olea europa*
Onion	*Allium cepa*
Orange	*Citrus sinensis*
Orpine (Eurasian Sedum)	*Sedum telephium*
Orrisroot (Florentine Iris)	*Iris florentina*
Paprika	*Capsicum annuum*
Parsley, Italian	*Petroselinum hortense*
Passionflower	*Passiflora incarnata*
Pedunculate Oak (English Oak)	*Quercus robur*
Peppermint	*Mentha piperita*
Periwinkle	*Vinca minor*
Plum (Garden Plum)	*Prunus domestica*
Pomegranate	*Punica granatum*
Pot Marigold (Calendula)	*Calendula officinalis*
Potato	*Solanum tuberosum*
Quack Grass	*Agropyron repens*
Quince	*Cydonia oblonga*
Radish	*Raphanus sativus*
Rampion	*Varianella olitoria*
Ransoms (Wild Garlic, Wood Garlic, Bear Garlic)	*Allium ursinum*
Raspberry (Common European Red)	*Rubus idaeus*
Restharow	*Ononis spinosa*
Rhubarb (Garden Rhubarb)	*Rheum rhabarbarum*
Roman Chamomile	*Chamaemelum nobile (Anthemis nobilis)*
Rose Bay Willow-Herb (Fireweed)	*Epilobium chamaenerium angustifolium*

Rosemary	*Rosmarinus officinalis*
Saffron	*Crocus sativus*
Sage	*Salvia officinalis*
Saint-John's-Wort	*Hypericum perforatum*
Samphire (Sea Fennel)	*Crithmum maritimum*
Sandalwood	*Santalum album*
Scotch Broom	*Cytisus scoparius*
Sea Fennel (Samphire)	*Crithmum maritimum*
Shave Grass	*Equisetum arvense*
Shepherd's Purse	*Capsella bursa-pastoris*
Silver Birch (European White Birch)	*Betula pendula*
Small Nettle (Dwarf Nettle)	*Urtica urens*
Sorrel (Garden Sorrel)	*Rumex acetosa*
Spinach	*Spinacia oleracea*
Summer Savory	*Satureja hortensis*
Sweet Marjoram (Knotted Marjoram)	*Origanum marjorana*
Sweet Flag (Calamus)	*Acorus calamus*
Sweet Clover (Melitot)	*Melilotus officinalis*
Tamarind	*Tamarindus indica*
Tarragon	*Artemisia dracunculus*
Teasel (Wild Teasel)	*Dipsacus sylvestris*
Thyme (Garden Thyme)	*Thymus vulgaris*
Tomato	*Lycopersicum esculentum*
Tormentil	*Potentilla erecta*
Turkish Boxwood	*Buxus sempervirens*
Valerian	*Valeriana officinalis*
Watercress	*Nasturtium officinale*
White Dead Nettle (Blind Nettle)	*Lamium album*
Whortleberry (Blueberry)	*Vaccinium myrtillus*
Wild Garlic (Wood Garlic, Bear's Garlic, Ransoms)	*Allium ursinum*
Wild Teasel (Teasel)	*Dipsacus sylvestris*
Wild Thyme (Creeping Thyme, Mother-of-Thyme)	*Thymus serpyllum*
Willow-Herb	*Epilobium montana*

Willow-Herb	*Epilobium roseum*
Willow	*Salix* species
Witch Grass (Couch Grass, Quack Grass)	*Agropyron repens*
Wood Sorrel	*Oxalis acetosella*
Wormwood (Absinthe)	*Artemisia absinthium*
Yarrow	*Achillea millefolium*

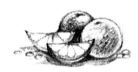

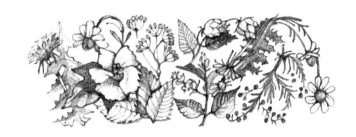

INDEX

L

labor contraction stimulation, for horses, 115
lack of appetite, 49
laryngitis, 39–40
Lavender–Arnica Vinegar, 73
Lemon Oil, 40
Lemon-Salt Gargle, 36
Lentil Juice Cure, 91
lice, in animals, 110
liver detoxification, 54
Lovage Tea, 105
Love Cream, 106
love potions, 103–106
low blood pressure, 46
lumbago, 92

M

make-up remover, 86
metabolism, stimulating, 62
Mistletoe–Black Elderberry Tea, 65
Mistletoe-Fennel Tea, 42
Mistletoe Wine, 49

N

neck wrinkles, 87
nervous heart condition, 45
nervous stress, 97–98
nervousness, 99–100
Nettle Juice–Yeast, 79
Nettle Tea, 73
Nettle Tincture, 70
Nine-Herb Fragrant Sleeping Pillow, 100

O

Oak Bark–Rose Tea, 57
obesity, in dogs, 112
Olive Leaf Tea, 44
Olive Oil–Lemon Juice Cure, 53
Onion Milk, 33
Orrisroot–English Ivy Tincture, 32
Orrisroot–Lungwort Tea, 29, 35
Oyster Shell Powder, 77

P

pain, rheumatic, 95–96
Paprika Honey, 52
parasites, of dogs, 112
Payos, 8
Peppermint–Rosemary Tincture, 79
persecution of Gypsies, 8
Pilar, 7–11
    healing art, 13–17
        See also specific ailments and recipes.
Pilar's Chest Tea, 31

Pilar's Cough Syrup, 37
Pilar's Diet for Rheumatism, 94–95
Pilar's Healthy Skin Diet, 80–81
Pilar's Love Potion, 105
Pilar's Poultice, 72
Pilar's Quince Compress, 87
Pilar's Rejuvenating Cream, 85
Pilar's Rheumatism Tea I, 93
Pilar's Rheumatism Tea II, 94
Pilar's Rosewater–Almond Milk Lotion, 86
Pilar's Spring Cure, 62
Pilar's Weight Loss Tea, 51
Pillow for Teething Children and Sick Adults, 101
Pine Resin Milk, 32
plants, botanical names, 117–123
Plum Jam, 60
Pomegranate Juice, 60
Potato Mask, 84
prostate problems, 69
psoriasis, 81
psychosomatic illnesses, 102
puffy skin, 84
purification of body, 51

Q

Quince Wine, 37

R

rabbits, remedies for, 112–113
rashes, skin, 77
recuperation from illness, for dogs, 111
rheumatism
    in horses, 115
    in humans, 89–91, 93–96
Rom, 8–9
Romani, 8–9
Root Juice, 75
Root Tea, 66
Rosemary–Sage–Red Wine Tonic, 25

S

Saint-John's-Wort Oil, 92
scabies, in animals, 110
sciatica, 92
Sea Fennel Tea, 69
sensuality, love potions and, 103–106
Seven Herb Tea, 101
shingles, 79
sinus infections, 39
skin
    blemishes, 77
    cleanser, 86
    nourishment of, 79